Cerebral Palsy:
From Diagnosis to Adult Life

Cerebral Palsy:
From Diagnosis to Adult Life

Peter Rosenbaum
and Lewis Rosenbloom

2012
Mac Keith Press

© 2012 Mac Keith Press

6 Market Road, London N7 9PW

Editor: Hilary M. Hart
Managing Director: Ann-Marie Halligan
Production Manager: Udoka Ohuonu
Project Management: Prepress Projects Ltd

First published in this edition 2012

British Library Cataloguing-in-Publication data
A catalogue record for this book is available from the British Library

Front cover shows Julia and Harrison Melluish. Photo reproduced with kind permission from Julia Melluish and is featured on the Peninsula Cerebral Research Unit for Childhood Disability Research (PenCRU) website (www.pencru.org). PenCRU carries out a broad programme of applied research that aims to improve the health and well-being of disabled children and their families.

ISBN: 978-1-908316-50-9

Typeset by Prepress Projects Ltd, Perth, UK

Printed by Henry Ling Limited, Dorchester, England
Mac Keith Press is supported by Scope

Contents

Authors

Peter Rosenbaum is a Professor of Paediatrics at McMaster University, Ontario, Canada, where he holds a Canada Research Chair in Childhood Disability, Mentoring and Dissemination. He is co-founder of the *CanChild* Centre for Childhood Disability Research.

Lewis Rosenbloom has been a Consultant Paediatric Neurologist since 1971. He holds an honorary appointment to the Royal Liverpool Children's NHS Foundation Trust UK. His special clinical, teaching and research interests are in paediatric neurodisability. He has published widely on many aspects of cerebral palsy including feeding issues and life expectation in disabled people.

Acknowledgements

We are very appreciative of the help and advice we have received from our families and from many friends and colleagues as we have attempted to distil and communicate our experiences. We would identify particularly Chris Verity, John Mantovani, Suzanne Shulman, Eileen Kinley and Toby Rosenbloom for their invaluable contributions. We are also grateful to Udoka Ohuonu and other colleagues from Mac Keith Press for their guidance and support throughout.

Foreword

When I joined the American Academy for Cerebral Palsy and Developmental Medicine (AACPDM) in 1984, it was in the hope of expanding my understanding of the care of children with neurodevelopmental disabilities (in those days termed 'handicaps'). As a freshly-minted child neurologist I had received a superb introduction to the scientific and clinical aspects of my craft with a who's who of late 20th century child neurology – Dodge, DeVivo, Fishman, Volpe – but was searching for something more. I wanted to understand the dimensions of care beyond the pathophysiology and the diagnosis; I wanted to know how best to serve the needs of the children with cerebral palsy and other neurodevelopmental conditions that I was seeing in my practice. That care, I felt, needed to be based on a deeper understanding of the human and relational aspects of the conditions themselves as well as the potential for meaningful therapeutic interventions for these patients and families. In short, I wanted to know what to do *after* I made the diagnosis. How should I communicate the diagnostic information; what interventions should I recommend; how should I judge the value of post-diagnostic interventions and, critically, how might I involve the patient and family in the treatment and caring process? To that end I sought a wider perspective of practice and a professional association with others interested in similar issues.

In that search, I found colleagues within the AACPDM who were seeking answers to such questions and who were discussing and researching ways to improve what we could offer our patients. Two of the very best of that group were Peter Rosenbaum and Lewis Rosenbloom. Therefore, I was delighted when my respected colleagues and friends asked me to read their manuscript about the very thing that had brought us together many years ago: understanding the multidimensional aspects of cerebral palsy, the prototypical childhood-onset disability. Having done so, I can heartily recommend the book.

The authors have produced a unique and valuable work by refracting the light of their clinical and teaching experience, research contributions and editorial leadership through the prism of a deep understanding and commitment to what matters most to the children and families we serve.

In this volume Professor Rosenbaum and Dr Rosenbloom aim to provide an understanding of cerebral palsy from multiple perspectives, but it is not, in their own words, a 'didactic treatment of the biomedical or epidemiological implications of cerebral palsy'. They have set themselves the task of speaking directly to families of children with cerebral palsy with the conviction that the family's and patient's concerns are the optimal focus of the service provider's interest. The authors' approach intermingles factual information with broader contextual interpretation and adds personal opinion where appropriate to provide a most useful perspective.

In dividing the book into four sections, the authors provide the opportunity for readers to focus on individual aspects of understanding. The first section provides basic information on the updated definition of cerebral palsy and current perspectives on its epidemiology, causation, classification and relationship to other neurological disabilities. The second section could easily stand alone as an educational primer on contextual factors in childhood disability. Separate chapters provide an erudite introduction to evidence-based critical appraisal methodology, the International Classification of Function, Disability and Health and a broad view of family issues. These discussions give the reader a framework for interpreting and conceptualizing research, structuring interventions most meaningfully and establishing communication to build therapeutic partnerships most effectively. The third section includes excellent contributions from Dr Margaret Mayston and covers diagnosis and assessment and the many aspects of therapeutic intervention planning, implementation and monitoring. The final section details the multilayered concepts of determining and measuring outcomes for individuals with cerebral palsy, a discussion on quality of life issues, a chapter on the process of transition to adulthood and a final chapter relating specifically to adults with cerebral palsy.

In the Preface, the authors describe their work as 'the culmination of dialogue and sharing of ideas as we have pursued issues and striven to understand cerebral palsy over many years'. Their commitment to both dialogue and sharing of ideas is clearly evident in the style and approach they choose. It is easy to recognize the authors' voices in the narrative and to hear their points of view coloured by the compassion and wisdom that come from decades in the clinic. The tone is relaxed and the information comes at a pace that enhances understanding of how the many pieces of this puzzle called cerebral palsy fit together – all premised on the understanding that we are talking about children and families. Reading this book is a comfortable and illuminating experience. Read it and you will think differently about cerebral palsy and how it affects your children, your patients and your fellow human beings.

John F. Mantovani
Chair, Department of Pediatrics, Mercy Children's Hospital;
Associate Professor, Clinical Neurology and Pediatrics, Washington University
School of Medicine,
St Louis, MO, USA

Preface

Readers of this handbook may find it useful to understand the perspectives from which we have conceived and written this book. We are experienced, developmentally trained clinicians with longstanding professional interests in cerebral palsy (CP) and other neurodevelopmental conditions. Our interests and perspectives are complementary: Lewis Rosenbloom has spent his career as a paediatric neurologist and mentor, while Peter Rosenbaum is a developmental paediatrician, teacher and researcher. We are also lifelong friends who have worked and learned together for several decades. This book represents the culmination of years of shared dialogue and ideas as we have pursued an understanding of issues surrounding CP.

In presenting our views we are relying not only on what we have learned in professional practice but also on the available research evidence. So far as the latter is concerned, we include our views on how evidence can be obtained, interpreted and utilized. We recognize that some of the details regarding particular assessments, measures, therapies and treatments will become dated, sooner or later. We celebrate the idea that new research constantly moves the field forward. We have therefore offered perspectives on how readers can become 'critical appraisers' of evidence, in order to have the skills to evaluate claims about any aspect of the story of CP, be it causation, the effectiveness of interventions or life-course trajectories for children and young people with CP.

We have chosen as our point of departure to address issues that we know to be of concern to families of children with CP – questions that obviously also concern front-line professionals. This emphasis differs somewhat from a didactic treatment of the biomedical or epidemiological implications of CP as a 'neurodevelopmental disability'. Rather, we propose to focus on the issues that challenge parents – the things that we as service providers can address together with parents and young people with CP. We hope that this approach will offer a primarily 'clinical' orientation that front-line health professionals, parents and other service providers will find useful.

The book is divided into four parts. In Part 1, Cerebral Palsy – Background Perspectives, we discuss CP as a clinical and epidemiological entity. The five chapters address what CP is, the epidemiology of CP, what we know about causation, how people talk about and categorize CP, and how CP relates to other neurodevelopmental disabilities.

Part 2, Contextual Factors and Critical Thinking, provides readers with an understanding of how we think, and how we hope others will think, about CP and related conditions. We both believe that an understanding of the research evidence is important. For this reason we have provided a primer on 'critical appraisal' that we hope will alert readers to the need to be analytically critical and thoughtful in assessing both conventional and new 'evidence' as it becomes available. Here we also present and briefly discuss two important concepts that should guide clinical practice. These are the World Health Organization's International Classification of Functioning, Disability and Health (ICF), including an illustrative case example, and an overview of the role of the family as the centrally important force in the lives of children with CP and other neurodevelopmental conditions.

In Part 3 we offer clinical perspectives in CP. Topics include clinical recognition and diagnosis of CP, comprehensive evaluation, principles and aims of intervention, and discussion about specific issues concerning interventions, both conventional and alternative. Readers seeking a detailed understanding of specific therapies, educational approaches and services are referred to appropriate resources that are beyond the scope of these discussions.

The final component of the book is Part 4, Outcomes in Childhood and Beyond. Here we provide a general discussion of 'outcomes'; we consider the challenges and opportunities associated with the transition to adulthood, and we remind readers that although CP begins as a 'children's condition', children with CP grow up to be adults with CP, and much remains to be learned and applied for the benefit of that adult population.

Throughout this book, but particularly with respect to Part 3, we have involved our colleague Margaret Mayston in our discussions. Margaret is both a physiotherapist and an academic and has contributed the majority of the chapter on issues in intervention. We are very grateful to her for her help. We also appreciate the help provided by Niina Kolehmainen in updating an earlier version of Chapter 2 on the epidemiology of CP.

It is appropriate that we comment on what are commonly described as the contrasting medical and social 'models' of disability present in modern society. In its pure form, the biomedical model perceives the disabled person as having a condition and being in need of treatment. It is said that this emphasizes a culture of dependency and that the methods of bringing about change for disabled people lie within the medical and associated professions.

By contrast, the social model concentrates on the person as a valued member of a diverse society. This approach suggests that the person with a disability is a unique individual who has the right to the same opportunities in life as anyone else. According to this model, the solution to 'disability' is to bring about attitudinal, environmental and organizational changes within present-day society.

Our perspective, illustrated by advocating the underlying philosophy and use of the International Classification of Functioning, Disability and Health (Chapter 7) and the central role of the family (Chapter 8), is that professionals working in the field of disability have moved on from what we have perceived to be as occasionally pejorative and conflicting approaches. Needless to say, we see these perspectives to be complementary, and hope that readers will agree that both are essential.

Terminology in our field continues to evolve. Whereas many people advocate the use of 'person first' language ('the individual with a disability'), others, including the authors, prefer 'disabled person' to reflect the social construction of disability as an interaction between the person and the environment, such that people may be 'disabled' when environmental factors limit their capacity for full engagement in life.

Another problem with terminology is the use of the terms 'mental retardation', 'cognitive impairment', '(severe) learning difficulties' and 'developmental retardation'. Although mental retardation is used in Diagnostic and Statistical Manual of Mental Disorders, 4th edition it is not a term that is acceptable or used by many clinicians. Common practice, and we have followed this, is to use the term developmental retardation for young children and either cognitive impairment or learning difficulties, which may be described as severe, in older children.

This book is dedicated to parents who find themselves on the path of an unexpected 'career', raising a child with CP; to adults with CP who are challenging us to recognize their life issues; and to the wide range of service provider colleagues who serve as families' guides on this journey. We have tried to speak to all equally, and hope that the ideas herein will resonate with all readers interested in CP across the lifespan.

Peter Rosenbaum, Hamilton, Ontario, Canada
Lewis Rosenbloom, Liverpool, UK
December 2011

Part 1

Cerebral palsy – background perspectives

Chapter 1

What is cerebral palsy?

Overview

The newly crafted definition and classification of cerebral palsy (CP) represent an international effort to bring coherence to an aspect of childhood neurodevelopmental disability that has often been associated with rather imprecise thinking. This chapter discusses the details of this definition to highlight what we believe are key concepts regarding CP. Whether the current efforts will prove to be more useful than the earlier systems remains to be seen. The authors hope that people will use this definition and classification across clinical and geographical boundaries, thus moving the field forward using consistent concepts and terminology.

In clinical medicine there is a longstanding tradition of labelling and categorizing diseases and disorders. It is always felt to be important to separate conditions based on a combination of factors such as their clinical features (e.g. presentation, manifestations, natural history), their biomedical underpinnings (derived from varied investigations) and even their responses to interventions. The process of diagnosis is important to both physicians and patients, because knowing what 'it' is helps us all to focus our attention on the 'right' condition (and also to know what 'it' is not.).

Any group of professionals working in the field of childhood disability will each have their own working definition of CP. None will be identical but all will have common components, and our aim is to synthesize these various working definitions. Morris (2007) has considered the historical perspectives and definitions of CP, and the interested reader should make reference to his helpful summary.

In the summer of 2004, an international group of clinicians and researchers gathered for 2 days in Bethesda, MD, USA, to consider one of the perennial questions in the field of developmental disability. For the past 40 years, the definition of CP had been the classic 1964 statement that CP is 'a disorder of movement and posture due to a defect or lesion of the immature brain' (Bax 1964). Despite some modest but useful enhancement of these ideas by Mutch et al. in 1992 (CP is 'an umbrella term covering a group of non-progressive, but often changing, motor impairment syndromes second-ary to lesions or anomalies of the brain arising in the early stages of development'), there remained uncertainty about both these specific definitions and, more generally, whether the term 'CP' had outlived its usefulness (Bax et al. 2007).

This 2004 meeting was jointly sponsored by the Castang Foundation of the UK and the United Cerebral Palsy Research and Educational Foundation of the USA. It was recognized that a host of factors in many fields of the clinical and biological sciences had increased our understanding of developmental neurobiology. The classic 'develop-mental disability' known as CP remains prevalent across the developed world, at a rate of 2–2.5 per 1000 people, and the rates are often rather higher in the developing world. For this reason, a reassessment of the concept and definition of CP was considered to be a useful undertaking.

The new definition, published in its final version in 2007, reads as follows:

> Cerebral palsy (CP) describes a group of permanent disorders of the develop-ment of movement and posture, causing activity limitation, that are attributed to non-progressive disturbances that occurred in the developing fetal or infant brain. The motor disorders of cerebral palsy are often accompanied by distur-bances of sensation, perception, cognition, communication, and behaviour, by epilepsy, and by secondary musculoskeletal problems.
>
> Rosenbaum et al. (2007)

The authors of this book contributed to this definition. We believe that there is still a place for differentiation of the idea of 'CP' as a clinical entity and as a 'diagnosis' (Rosenbloom 2007). For these reasons we will offer some thoughts about the ways in which this set of ideas may inform thinking not only about CP but about conditions across the spectrum of developmental disabilities.

We consider that it is important to examine the thinking behind the new defini-tion and offer personal reflections and perspective. We argue that this revised and expanded definition may help people to understand the challenges inherent in trying to define conditions that are as much conceptual and phenomenological notions as they are biomedical entities. We also discuss some of the 'rough edges' of the concept of 'CP'.

To illustrate these concepts, the early histories of two children with CP are briefly recounted. This is to emphasize that children with CP have varied early histories and frequently have more than just a motor disorder.

Child 1

AA was born at 37 weeks' gestation. There was evidence of maternal hypertension and of restricted fetal growth in the later part of gestation. Labour commenced spontaneously, and during its course there was evidence of suboptimal fetal status from a pathological cardiotocograph trace and acidosis on fetal scalp sampling. Delivery was by emergency Caesarean section.

The infant's birthweight and head circumference were between the third and tenth centiles. There was cardiorespiratory depression at the time of birth and depressed Apgar scores for the first 10 minutes in spite of prompt resuscitation. Thereafter there was a neonatal encephalopathy with seizures.

During the course of her first 2 years it became apparent that there was slow development of motor abilities, social responsiveness and language. There was uncertainty about visual functioning. There was slowing of head growth, with the circumference falling to below the third centile. Magnetic resonance brain imaging demonstrated extensive acquired white matter signal change in the cerebral hemispheres.

On examination at the age of 2 years, AA presented with a bilateral motor disorder considered to be CP. Motor skills were best classified as being Gross Motor Function Classification System (GMFCS) level V (Palisano et al. 2008) (the full GMFCS is reproduced in Appendix I). Muscle tone was primarily increased, with spasticity affecting all four limbs. Her weight was below the third centile and oral feeding was difficult and prolonged. Overall, a delay in development was confirmed.

AA's history illustrates the need to recognize the relationship between her brain damage and the circumstances of gestation and labour, to appreciate that her disabilities extend way beyond her impairments of motor function and to deal with the implications of her need for lifetime care.

Child 2

BB was born at term after an uneventful gestation, labour and delivery. His birthweight and head size were close to the 50th centile and the neonatal period was uneventful.

At age 7 months he had a preference for using his left arm. By the time he was starting to stand at 14 months, it was evident that there was increased muscle tone in the right leg. He walked independently at age 15 months and was considered to have a right hemiparesis. Magnetic resonance brain imaging demonstrated focal infarction within the territory of the left middle cerebral artery.

At age 9 years he functions at GMFCS level I, and there is evidence of significant right-sided calf muscle hypertonus: he weight-bears on his toes on the right foot during walking. He is reluctant to use the right arm and hand, and is classified as functioning at level II on the Manual Ability Classification System (MACS) (Eliasson et al. 2006) (the full MACS is reproduced in Appendix II).

There is also concern because his educational progress is uneven, he has some behavioural difficulties and he has had two seizures.

Here the issues for consideration principally relate to understanding the significance of the totality of his motor impairments for independence and adult functioning, and to appreciate that his prognosis in these fields may be adversely affected by cognitive and behavioural difficulties and by epilepsy.

With these case illustrations as background, we present some issues that we believe should be considered when we talk about CP, and certainly when professionals engage in the assessment and management of children and young people with CP.

Should cerebral palsy be considered a 'disease', a 'diagnosis', a 'developmental disorder' or a simply a 'condition'?

The first issue that requires consideration is the question of whether CP should be considered a 'disease', a 'diagnosis', a 'developmental disorder' or simply a 'condition'. In so far as CP is known to be associated with a host of proven aetiological factors (e.g. brain malformations, kernicterus, maternal iodine deficiency) and established risk factors (e.g. preterm birth, being a twin, maternal genital tract infections, perinatal adversity), it seems clear that CP is not a single 'disease' in the way that type I diabetes or Duchenne muscular dystrophy might be so labelled. With today's sensitive imaging techniques it is increasingly apparent that the nature, timing and distribution of brain impairments are all very varied and that the 'clinical–pathological' (in this case clinical–radiological) correlations are also varied and often distinct. Work by Bax and colleagues (2006) in a large European study of CP has shown that there are important relationships between the location of brain impairments (as identified by expert interpretation of magnetic resonance scans) and what might be called clinical 'syndromes' involving both motor function impairments and a host of other neurodevelopmental difficulties.

Given both the widely varying manifestations of CP and the many causal pathways thought to be important in its genesis (Stanley et al. 2000), the idea of referring to CP as a 'disease' seems somewhat problematic. What does a 'diagnosis' of CP mean? As outlined by any of the traditional definitions presented at the start of this chapter, the term describes impairment in the development of motor function and posture presenting early in life. Leaving aside for a moment the specific question of what 'early' means, it must be emphasized that all these definitions refer to aspects of a child's gross motor development rather than to any specific biomedical marker by which the diagnosis can be confirmed or ruled out.

Although we argue that diagnosis is less precise in CP than in conditions with a discrete biomedical 'cause', it is certainly important to reach the formulation that this child has 'CP', to assess that child carefully as outlined elsewhere in this book, to communicate the findings empathically to the family, to plan and review interventions and to follow the child's development on a long-term basis.

There is often debate about how soon one can be comfortable about the 'diagnosis'. Some argue that one cannot be certain that a child has CP before the age of 2 years, while others (including the authors) believe that in many cases – usually in those whose functional manifestations are more apparent ('severe') – one can identify and at least tentatively label the patterns of aberrant motor posture and function at 6 months of age or sometimes even sooner. Certainly a realistic approach for clinicians is to be prepared to identify and act on 'variations' in a child's early motor development that compromise functional development (Rosenbaum 2006a,b). This can be done when there are problems with 'quantity' and/or 'quality' of motor behaviour by referring the infant or young child to the appropriate developmental services while continuing to follow the child's progress. This should be done, among other activities, in order to evaluate the natural history of the child's development and eventually to decide whether the child's status actually fits the definition of 'CP'. As Weindling (2008) has pointed out, it follows that it is difficult to predict CP at a presymptomatic level from, for example, the presence of abnormalities on neonatal cranial ultrasound studies. We support the ideas contained in the 2007 definition of CP that there should be some evidence of 'activity limitation' and not simply risk factors or the presence of isolated 'impairments' (problems in body structure – see Chapter 7) such as may be found in people with CP.

The excellent Surveillance of Cerebral Palsy in Europe (SCPE) group (Cans 2000) has offered one epidemiologically motivated compromise. Members of the many CP registries that contribute to this database make a tentative ascertainment of CP at any age, but only when the child has passed his or her fourth birthday will the SCPE members confirm for their register that the child has the clinical findings of CP, as outlined in their very useful manual (SCPE Reference and Training Manual). They argue that after age 4 years it should be clear whether the child's earlier-identified functional problems have disappeared or whether they have progressed in ways that are phenomenologically inconsistent with the definition of CP. In the interim, of course, one would expect such children to be carefully monitored and their families offered appropriate developmental interventions, few of which are specific to CP.

What are the implications of considering cerebral palsy as a 'developmental disability'?

What we believe to be the most significant contribution to the new definition of CP are the ideas contained in the second sentence (see p. 4). It is here that the various potential disorders of *function*, in addition to the 'motor' manifestations, have been formally identified as part of the spectrum of the CP picture. There is no implication that these functional difficulties are *necessarily* part of the condition (although frequently they are observed), but by explicitly including them the authors of the new definition have endeavoured to focus attention on the fact that many aspects of a child's development *may* be associated with and impacted upon by 'CP', both primarily (as part of the impairment in brain structure and function) as well as secondarily (related to developmental challenges associated with the limitations in motor function).

The terminology in the newly crafted definition of CP highlights the *impact* of the condition on a child's development, function and life trajectory as opposed to emphasizing solely the brain malfunction or 'disease' components of CP. This approach directly leads to thinking about CP (and many other early-onset childhood problems) in terms of how it actually or potentially alters the patterns of a child's development. This idea distinguishes the important biomedical aspects of CP or other developmental conditions (e.g. issues of diagnosis, aetiology, genetic implications, 'treatments', etc.) from the challenges associated with 'management' and life-course perspectives.

Among these challenges is the question of the extent to which one 'treats' CP by addressing the primary 'impairments' associated with it (e.g. spasticity, hypertonicity, abnormalities of reflex function) and the extent to which one works to promote functional capability with techniques and equipment that may include 'augmentative and alternative' interventions. These latter interventions, when provided at developmentally appropriate times to accommodate children's emerging interests in those aspects of function, may allow children to be functional despite the fact that progress is atypical, and despite the reality that the underlying neurological impairments may not be altered by these interventions. (Of course, when impairment-directed treatments such as botulinum toxin are indicated to moderate the effects of spasticity they should also be applied for the appropriate indications, without assuming that their use will, by themselves, necessarily change function [Wright et al. 2008].)

Butler's work (Butler et al. 1984; Butler 1986) illustrates the value of alternative interventions in enhancing function and development. She demonstrated the remarkable influence that powered ('augmented') mobility had on children as young as 2 years and 6 months of age. The children's language, exploration, social function and even their efforts at self-initiated movement were all profoundly impacted when they were provided with an external means to move. Control of powered mobility was something they learned to do independently within a relatively small number of hours of exposure and practice. This intervention did not address the basic impairments at all. Rather, it represented an 'environmental' manipulation that impacted upon the children's lives in ways that no currently known 'treatments' could possibly do (Rosenbaum 2008). This work anticipated by almost 20 years the current ideas inherent in the World Health Organization's International Classification of Functioning, Disability and Health (ICF) (World Health Organization 2001), about which more is written later in this book (see Chapter 7).

At the same time, it must be noted that there are still many traditional 'orthodox' impairment-based treatments that eschew the use of alternative interventions, such as walkers for mobility or sign language for communication of children with hearing or language impairments. The proponents of these approaches seem to want to direct therapeutic efforts exclusively at remediating the underlying impairment in order to promote 'normal' function. We argue that such thinking is excessively conservative in scope. It is unsupported by sound clinical research to bolster the thesis that promoting 'normal' function is a better approach than the more eclectic one recommended here, nor is there convincing evidence that it is even possible to 'correct' biomedical impairments in ways that make a functional difference, thereby making it the right course of action to take.

The concept of cerebral palsy as a life-long condition

The third issue to highlight in the definition – implicit in the word 'permanent' in the first sentence of the new definition – is the concept that CP is a life-long condition. Like virtually all 'neurodevelopmental' disorders, CP has traditionally been thought of as a 'childhood disease'. This is understandable in so far as CP and related neuro-developmental conditions present in the very early years of life, and have always been recognized and managed within the child health systems of most countries. The reality, of course, is that mortality associated with these conditions is now very low (Strauss et al. 2007), and the vast majority of children with CP become adults with CP. Indeed, there are more adults with CP than children with CP. This challenging fact has impor-tant implications for people who have traditionally thought primarily or exclusively about 'childhood' disabilities.

Among the important realities is that in most parts of the world adult-focused ser-vices are unfamiliar with these 'childhood conditions'. While CP is often superficially similar to stroke, acquired brain injury and other neuromotor disorders experienced by adults, people with CP bring to adulthood a life-long experience of development that is fundamentally different from that of people who have lived conventional lives until an adult condition interfered with their function. One of the implications of this difference is that people working in adult services may have little or no appreciation of these unusual life trajectories and 'cultures', and may be ill equipped to help adults with CP to fit in to the adult world.

It is also the case that the medical aspects of the lives of people with CP are often much less important than the social, vocational and community-living dimensions for which adults with CP need support. Underemployment and social isolation are often identified as key challenges for adults with CP and other neurodevelopmental disabili-ties – but the social and counselling services available to adults with CP are usually grossly inadequate in helping them. At the same time, there are important aspects of the processes of ageing with CP that need to be much better understood in order not to assume that anything that happens to an adult with CP can be ascribed simply to their underlying 'childhood' neuromotor condition (O'Brien and Rosenbloom 2009).

Another consideration regarding the adult component of the CP story is really a corol-lary of the first two – namely that traditional therapy efforts directed at the mobility and related 'motor' function dimensions of CP are much too narrowly focused to address life-course issues. If one sees CP as both a neurodevelopmental disorder and a permanent condition – as the new definition emphasizes – then it is essential that we reframe our goals for 'therapy', 'treatment' and 'management' during childhood to address the *developmental* implications of these conditions and that we focus our inter-ventions to ensure that they are developmentally appropriate. This means grounding all our interventions within a broader canvas of life trajectories of children, working towards promoting functional abilities and a sense of competence and capability, taking a strengths-based approach rather than continuing the tradition of cataloguing what disabled children cannot do. It also emphasizes the importance of continuity of thought and action across the lifespan to create seamless services as young people with CP move into the adult world.

The final implication of these ideas is, of course, that interventions should always be carried out within a family-centred service focus. Beyond the lip-service acknowledgement that most child health professionals would easily pay to this idea is the reality that parents need to be helped to understand that their child with CP has a 'developmental' challenge rather than perceive them solely as a child with a 'disease' (produced by 'brain damage') that must be 'treated'. Parents need to be well informed about management options, and they need to be listened to with respect to their goals for their child's development. An important randomized clinical trial from the Netherlands by Ketelaar and her colleagues (2001) showed powerfully that interventions directed at addressing parent- and child-identified functional goals led to better long-term functional outcomes than traditional impairment-based therapies – and with less intervention.

'Rough edges' in the definition of cerebral palsy

A fourth issue inherent in the new definition of CP is that there continue to be some 'rough edges' – those areas that remained controversial at the end of the 2004 consensus meeting. One question concerns the upper limit of the timing of 'disturbances that occurred in the developing fetal or infant brain' (Rosenbaum 2007). Children may acquire impairments of the central nervous system after birth owing to events as varied as brain trauma, central nervous system infections, asphyxia and cerebral malaria (in developing countries). The issue of the upper limit of the timing of causal events is perennially perplexing. This is true in part because from an epidemiological perspective it is important to frame the scope of the events that might be associated with the outcome 'CP' and might be relevant to the varied causal pathways that are being identified as potentially important to the genesis of CP. On the other hand, from a clinical and health services perspective, the identification, management and long-term follow-up of children with either early ('congenital') CP or so-called late CP ('acquired' in the first couple of years in the young developing child) should be similar and should focus on the 'developmental' aspects of this quintessentially 'neurodevelopmental' condition as these concern children and families.

Another element of the definition that has provoked considerable discussion over the years concerns the notion of 'non-progressive' disturbances. The issue is complicated in at least three important ways. Children with CP naturally change and develop over time, so that virtually all aspects of their lives and function may look different at different ages. Understanding the natural history of these changes and developments is important in order to distinguish 'disease progression' from 'change and development' inherent in childhood, even in the face of biological impairments that may constrain or inflect the patterns of developmental progress.

While there are classic neurodegenerative disorders of childhood that are clearly 'progressive', it may well be the case that some of the traditional, apparently 'static' encephalopathic conditions of infants and children are slowly 'progressive' in ways that have not previously been recognized. In addition, it seems likely that adults with CP age differently from other adults, related at least in part to factors such as 'wear and tear' on their systems, including the development of secondary conditions of muscles and joints. These accelerated changes in body structure and function may be associated with limitations in fitness imposed by challenges both intrinsic and extrinsic to people with CP (such as the paucity of community-based programmes and services available to these adults). If this is true then there may be important and as yet unrecognized opportunities for secondary prevention of the consequences of CP on adult well-being.

There appears to be no easy answer to this question about 'progressive' conditions, but the annotation accompanying the new definition states clearly: 'Motor dysfunction which results from recognized progressive brain disorders is not considered CP.' Clinical examples might include ataxia telangiectasia or Rett syndrome, each of which can, in its early manifestations, resemble CP. The previously described SCPE approach to the formal ascertainment of children as having CP at the age of 4 years makes it possible in most cases to identify children whose developmental course reflects a progressive as opposed to static condition, and who by definition are considered not to have 'CP'. As noted earlier, the authors believe that at a clinical level one can and should identify, and offer help with, problems with a child's motor development, whatever the specific biomedical diagnosis. Whether and when to intervene to address and to help children experiencing impaired function constitutes a clinical decision separate from whether the problem is eventually labelled as 'CP'.

Another rough edge is the challenge associated with motor impairments in an affected individual that are considered modest or even subtle. At a diagnostic level, the question can then reasonably be raised as to whether it is still appropriate to use the term 'CP' to report the child's condition. There can be no dogmatic answer to this question, especially if features such as very refractory epilepsy or profound cognitive impairment dominate the clinical picture. In practice we are comfortable with still using the CP label when the motor impairments are clinically apparent, even though they may be functionally of limited importance, but we do recognize that this is a grey area.

Classification of cerebral palsy
Finally, it is appropriate to consider briefly the question of how to classify CP – an issue that the Bethesda group addressed in its 2004 deliberations and which is more fully discussed in Chapter 4. Several basic points were identified. First, classification may be done for one or more of several reasons: to describe a child or a population; to predict future status; or to evaluate change in function. Second, there is a host of dimensions on which classification can be done, so it is important to be clear what purpose(s) one has in mind before applying any specific system. For example, traditional clinical descriptors of CP have focused on (1) *topography* (which parts of the body are involved); (2) the nature of the *motor impairment(s)* (whether the motor system is stiff and 'spastic', loose and 'hypotonic' or experiences fluctuations in motor control – 'athetotic', 'ataxic' or

'dystonic'); and (3) *severity* (traditionally characterized as 'mild', 'moderate' or 'severe', whatever those words mean).

For any measurement system to be useful (and classification is a form of measurement), it must be both reliable (provide consistent answers across observers and time when status is stable) and valid (meaningful and a reflection of the 'truth'). It is important to note that few of the traditional classifications of CP have been shown to be either reliable or valid. Newer purpose-designed systems for people with CP have been created and validated for their ability to describe/discriminate both gross motor function (the GMFCS [Palisano et al. 1997, 2008]) and manual abilities (the MACS [Eliasson et al. 2006]). These systems (reproduced in Appendices I and II, respectively) are known to be acceptable to parents as well as service providers and researchers, and it has been shown repeatedly that the evaluations of parents and professionals are highly consistent with one another (Morris et al. 2004, 2006).

It was demonstrated by Gorter et al. (2004) not only that the GMFCS is the most (perhaps the only) reliable gross motor clinical classification system, but also that the various levels of the GMFCS each include children with a variety of topographic distributions and types of motor impairment. These latter characteristics overlap considerably with each other and seem to be unhelpful with respect to describing the *functional* aspects of a person's CP. Thus, once again, it is important to observe that whatever classification systems are chosen, they must meet identified needs and be sound measurement tools if they are to fulfil the purposes to which they are put. These issues are discussed in more detail in Chapter 4.

To conclude, we reiterate our belief that the concept 'CP' remains a useful one for both clinical and epidemiological purposes. In particular, this approach allows us to talk with and counsel parents and families, and people with CP, reasonably clearly about a defined group of motor impairment syndromes for which the aetiology, natural history, management and life outcomes are becoming increasingly understood. We believe that abandoning this term would be counterproductive to all concerned.

References

Bax MC (1964) Terminology and classification of cerebral palsy. *Dev Med Child Neurol* 11: 295–7.

Bax M, Tydeman C, Flodmark O (2006) Clinical and MRI correlates of cerebral palsy: the European Cerebral Palsy Study. *JAMA* 296:1602–8.

Bax MCO, Flodmark O, Tydeman C (2007) Definition and classification of cerebral palsy. From syndrome toward disease. *Dev Med Child Neurol* 49 (Suppl. 109): 39–41.

Butler C. (1986) Effects of powered mobility on self-initiated behaviors of very young children with locomotor disability. *Dev Med Child Neurol* 28: 325–32.

Butler C, Okamoto GA, McKay TM (1984) Motorized wheelchair driving by disabled children. *Arch Phys Med Rehabil* 65: 95–7.

Cans C (2000) Surveillance of cerebral palsy in Europe: a collaboration of cerebral palsy surveys and registers. *Dev Med Child Neurol* 42: 816–24.

Eliasson AC, Krumlinde Sundholm L et al. (2006) The Manual Ability Classification System (MACS) for children with cerebral palsy: scale development and evidence of validity and reliability. *Dev Med Child Neurol* 48: 549–54.

Gorter JW, Rosenbaum PL, Hanna SE et al. (2004) Limb distribution, type of motor disorder and functional classification of cerebral palsy: how do they relate? *Dev Med Child Neurol* 46: 461–7.

Ketelaar M, Vermeer A, Hart H, van Petegem-van Beek E, Helders PJ (2001) Effects of a functional therapy program on motor abilities of children with cerebral palsy. *Phys Ther* 81: 1534–45.

Morris C (2007) Definition and classification of cerebral palsy: a historical perspective. *Dev Med Child Neurol* 49 (Suppl. 109): 3–7.

Morris C, Galuppi BE, Rosenbaum PL (2004) Reliability of family report for the Gross Motor Function Classification System. *Dev Med Child Neurol* 46: 455–60.

Morris C, Kurinczuk JJ, Fitzpatrick R, Rosenbaum PL (2006) Who best to make the assessment? Professionals and families' classifications of gross motor function are highly consistent. *Arch Dis Child* 91: 675–9.

Mutch LW, Alberman E, Hagberg B, Kodama K, Velickovic MV (1992) Cerebral palsy epidemiology: where are we now and where are we going? *Dev Med Child Neurol* 34: 547–55.

O'Brien G, Rosenbloom L (2009) Developmental disability and ageing. In: O'Brien G and Rosenbloom L (eds) London: Mac Keith Press.

Palisano R, Rosenbaum P, Walter S, Russell D, Wood E, Galuppi B (1997) Development and validation of a gross motor function classification system for children with cerebral palsy. *Dev Med Child Neurol* 39: 214–23.

Palisano RJ, Rosenbaum P, Bartlett D, Livingston MH (2008) Content validity of the expanded and revised Gross Motor Function Classification System. *Dev Med Child Neurol* 50: 744–50.

Rosenbaum P (1986) Effects of powered mobility on self-initiated behaviours of very young children with locomotor disability. *Dev Med Child Neurol* 50: 644.

Rosenbaum P (2006a) The definition and classification of cerebral palsy: are we any further ahead in 2006? *NeoReviews* 7: e569–e574. Also available at: http://neoreviews.aappublications.org/cgi/content/full/7/11/e569.

Rosenbaum P (2006b) Classification of abnormal neurological outcome. *Early Hum Dev* 82: 167–71.

Rosenbaum, P (2008) Effects of powered mobility on self-initiated behaviours of very young children with locomotor disability. *Dev Med Child Neurol* 50: 644

Rosenbaum P, Paneth N, Leviton A, Goldstein M, Bax M (2007) Definition and classification document. In: The definition and classification of cerebral palsy. Baxter P (ed.) *Dev Med Child Neurol* 49 (Suppl. 2): 8–14.

Rosenbloom L (2007) Definition and classification of cerebral palsy. Definition, classification, and the clinician. *Dev Med Child Neurol* 49 (Suppl. 109): 43.

SCPE Reference and Training Manual. Available at: http://www-rheop.ujf-grenoble.fr/scpe2/site_scpe/index.php (accessed 25 March 2008).

Stanley FJ, Blair E, Alberman E (2000) *Cerebral Palsies: Epidemiology and Causal Pathways*. London: Mac Keith Press.

Strauss D, Shavelle R, Reynolds R, Rosenbloom L, Day S (2007) Survival in cerebral palsy in the last 20 years: signs of improvement? *Dev Med Child Neurol* 49: 86–92.

Weindling M (2008) Gross motor functional abilities and periventricular leukomalacia. *Dev Med Child Neurol* 50: 647.

World Health Organization (2001) *International Classification of Functioning, Disability and Health (ICF)*. Geneva: World Health Organization.

Wright FV, Rosenbaum PL, Goldsmith CH, Law M, Fehlings DL (2008) How do changes in body functions and structures, activity, and participation relate in children with cerebral palsy? *Dev Med Child Neurol* 50: 283–9.

Chapter 2
Epidemiology: patterns and causes of cerebral palsy

with Niina Kolehmainen

Overview

We begin this chapter with an overview of the concepts and methods that underlie epidemiological thinking and about which readers need to be aware of when they read epidemiological studies of cerebral palsy (CP) or any other chronic childhood condition.[a] We then illustrate from the wide range of published work on the epidemiology of CP some of the data that have become available and their significance for both clinical services and planning health policies and services, along with other provisions. We draw attention to the strengths and limitations of epidemiological work in this area of practice. We also comment on the value and limitations of follow-up population studies.

Epidemiology is the study of health and illness in a population. The epidemiology of CP can inform us about the distribution patterns in a community and possible causes, and about whether, over time, these patterns may be changing. Such information can help us to pinpoint factors that seem to be associated with a greater risk of developing CP. We can also learn whether there are changes in the number of new cases that are associated with changes in patterns of service delivery, such as regionalization of high-risk perinatal care or the introduction of new technical or other health service systems. To make use of the epidemiological evidence, it is important to understand the terms used, so these are outlined briefly below.[a]

---

a   Part of this text has been adapted from the following report: Missiuna C, Smits C, Rosenbaum P, Woodside J, Law P (2001) *The Prevalence of Childhood Disability: Facts and Issues.* A report prepared for the Ontario Ministry of Health and Long-term Care by *CanChild* Centre for Childhood Disability Research.

What is meant by 'prevalence' and 'incidence' of cerebral palsy?

Understanding patterns of CP involves, among other things, determining the number of people who have it. There are two common ways to establish and report this information. *Prevalence* refers to how many people in a defined population have CP at a specific point in time (e.g. the proportion of Canadians who had CP in 2010). To obtain a prevalence of CP, one assesses everyone within the defined population (or more often a representative 'sample' from which one can generalize to the whole population) and then counts how many people have CP within a particular time window. Prevalence is usually described as the 'number per thousand lives births' in the reference population.

Studies of prevalence enable us to identify whether the distribution of people with CP varies systematically on a geographical basis, perhaps as an indication that specific factors may be important in its genesis. Such a situation would arise, for example, when one identifies cases of CP in regions where iodine deficiency is endemic among women of childbearing age (Hong and Paneth 2008). Iodine deficiency predisposes their children to be born with hypothyroidism and a developmental disability syndrome that includes mental slowness, deafness and CP. Such information will be useful not only to scientists interested in identifying causal pathways in the development of CP, but also for policy-makers and community planners. For these latter individuals, it is essential to know how preventative and management services should be allocated across a region in order to maximize the benefit to the community in need of such services.

Incidence of CP refers to the number of *new* cases of CP that appear within a defined period of time (e.g. the number of Canadians diagnosed as having CP between 1 January 2010 and 31 December 2010). To calculate incidence of CP, one seeks out and counts all new cases that are identified in a specified time period (usually 1y). The incidence of CP is usually expressed as 'cases per thousand per year' (this allows standardization in the reporting of different conditions).

To measure the prevalence and incidence of any condition, a clear definition of that condition is crucial – one that can be used in practice to identify people who should be counted and to exclude people who should not. Variations in the definitions of what constitutes CP result in variations in the number of people identified as having it. Similarly, variations in methods of measuring or classifying CP may lead to very different estimates of either prevalence or incidence.

What is meant by 'diagnosis' in the context of cerebral palsy?

As discussed in Chapter 1, the definition of CP has changed over time. While there have been efforts to establish an agreed definition and to harmonize the use of that definition in practice, variations between countries continue to exist. For this reason some of the variation in the reported incidence and prevalence of CP may be attributable to the challenges related to making the diagnosis of CP.

Neurodevelopmental conditions like CP differ from some specific biomedical conditions with respect to the basis on which a diagnosis is made. It is much easier to make an accurate and specific diagnosis of some neurodevelopmental conditions than others. The basis on which, in general, diagnoses are made can be summarized as follows:

1   A consistent biological 'marker' (e.g. a specific detectable genetic abnormality) may indicate the presence of a specific 'disease' (Bradley et al. 1993) or condition (e.g. Down syndrome). In these situations, it is relatively simple to make a diagnosis (e.g. the child either has or does not have Down syndrome, based on having or not having trisomy 21).
2   In some readily recognizable conditions (e.g. Tourette syndrome), no specific 'marker' has yet been identified that would allow the diagnosis to be established with certainty using laboratory tests (Mason et al. 1998). Nonetheless, the syndromic pattern is evident and reasonably consistent across time and space.
3   The way the child presents (for example clinically, or in their behaviour and abilities as reported by those close to the child) often indicates the presence of a collection of difficulties that have common features, although these may be extremely variable. Autism and CP are two such conditions that are defined phenomenologically.

Thus, when considering the prevalence literature, it is important to identify whether one is talking about a specific 'disease' with a known and detectable 'marker' that distinguishes and validates the diagnosis, or a 'disorder' for which the underlying biological 'causes' are either unknown or vary from one person to another. The processes of ascertainment and validation of these different categories will clearly vary from one situation to another.

The diagnosis of CP is based on the way the child presents (Rosenbaum et al. 2007). The diagnosis is described and defined by clinical features, which include the behaviour and abilities of the child (see Chapter 1 for the definition), and there may be a wide variety of underlying impairments that produce varied clinical patterns that are recognized as belonging to CP.

A consensus recently reached on the definition and classification of CP has allowed for a more consistent use of the diagnosis. In parallel with this development, there has been a remarkable collaboration of surveys and registers across eight countries in Europe, combining them into what is now a single database (Cans 2000). However, a certain amount of judgement continues to be required in deciding whether an individual does or does not have CP. While the measurement and classification of CP have improved over time, many instruments with unknown reliability and validity are still used. It is therefore important for any reader of the literature to seek clarity about the terms and methods that were used to identify and diagnose those with the condition.

How is the 'severity' of a condition described?
Among the many challenges of estimating issues such as incidence and prevalence of a condition is the problem of describing and reporting its severity. This is especially problematic at the least-affected end of the spectrum as it is almost always easier to find 'severe' cases of a condition than those that are more 'mild'. (This is true because

when a child's difficulties are 'severe' there is a far higher likelihood that people will recognize the presence of the condition and agree upon how to label it.)

Reporting the severity of a condition involves making judgements about (1) the factors on which severity is measured and (2) the threshold at which it is considered 'severe'. In children with CP, the severity of their difficulties can be considered in relation to at least three factors (World Health Organization 2007): the degree of impairment in body structure and function (e.g. damage at the level of nervous system); the range of activities that the child struggles to do (e.g. limitations of abilities and skills); and the restrictions on the child's participation in life (e.g. restricted involvement in play and educational pursuits).

Defining the severity of a child's CP is likely to depend on the point of view adopted. Defining severity from a medical point of view (e.g. as a degree of impairment in body structure and function) may result in a very different conclusion than considering severity from the perspective of the parent or the child (e.g. the degree of problems in participating in daily activities, or the stress that caring for a child with difficulties places on family life). Furthermore, CP is often a multifaceted condition and may be associated with coexisting conditions (Boyle et al. 1994) (so-called 'comorbidity'). These are likely to further influence the severity of the child's medical problems and participation difficulties, and it is important to consider this 'combined severity' when investigating the child and families' healthcare needs, service utilization, perceived health status, school performance and attendance, etc.

In studies of prevalence and incidence of CP, it is always important to understand how the severity of the condition was defined, what classification systems were used to describe the difficulties experienced by the children included in the study and how coexisting conditions and difficulties were recognized and taken into account. One's confidence in the data presented in any given study will increase when, among other design features, standardized, reliable and valid classification systems have been applied appropriately. To date, there are two systems that have been shown to be reliable and valid in classifying the severity of gross motor abilities (Palisano et al. 1997, 2008) and fine motor/manual ability (Eliasson et al. 2006) in children with CP – the Gross Motor Function Classification System and the Manual Ability Classification System, respectively . These instruments also provide excellent examples of how clinical classification systems can be applied to bridge the gap between clinical and epidemiological perspectives on CP. (Issues of classification of CP, including a discussion of levels of functional capacity, are elaborated in some detail in Chapter 4.)

When can childhood disabilities like cerebral palsy be detected?
Different childhood disabilities can be detected at different stages of the child's development. Some are evident at or even before birth, for example congenital disorders such as Down syndrome, spina bifida and cleft lip and palate are present and recognizable at the time of birth and increasingly by ultrasound assessments done during pregnancy. Others may become evident ('emerge') more slowly, and may only become apparent

when a child fails to reach typical milestones (e.g. the gross motor difficulties of a child with emerging CP) or with the appearance of unusual behaviours (e.g. stereotypical behaviours and social difficulties in a child with emerging autism).

The variable pattern and timing of the emergence of disabilities obviously has an important impact on what constitutes evidence of any given condition within the childhood disability spectrum. This pattern influences the likelihood with which a condition may be detected at a specific age, and thus has an impact on the age(s) at which evidence about the presence of a condition should be collected for epidemiological purposes.

For conditions diagnosed on the basis of the clinical (functional) presentation of the child, one can only be certain that the child has 'it' once the child's history and assessment show a clear pattern that fits the definition of the condition of interest. The definition for CP (see Chapter 1) states that, to meet the diagnostic criteria, the child must have a disorder of the development of movement and posture associated with activity limitations. An assessment of whether or not a child has these difficulties relies on comparing his or her performance against what is known about the typical development of children. This comparison can be difficult as typical development in itself varies considerably among children. For that reason, many people would, for example, be reluctant to apply a firm and specific diagnosis of 'CP' as opposed to other developmental motor problems or even variations of typical development before 6 to 12 months of age (although again there will be an inverse relationship between severity and age at recognition and formal labelling of the condition). The clinical pictures of these conditions are often quite fluid and relatively undifferentiated in early development.

One example of this issue has been reported by Kuban et al. (2008). Their approach to the assessment of motor development in 2-year-old children was to develop a decision tree (an 'algorithm') for detecting CP. It is based on a small number of motor function items, and certainly may identify children with impaired motor function. However, as the authors themselves note, the criterion standard 'diagnosis' of CP still relies on an expert's clinical evaluation. We believe that what is being identified by the Kuban et al. algorithm is children with motor development difficulties that *may* be CP but might of course be a reflection of other conditions and disorders that can only be formally ascertained by clinical assessment. They may equally be manifestations of variations in early motor development that eventually appear to be typical rather than 'abnormal' function (Rosenbaum 2006).

In interpreting the findings from epidemiological studies of CP, it is critical to consider how the study sampling and recruitment methods have taken into consideration the natural history of CP. It is also important to keep in mind that the older a child is, the more likely he or she is to come to the attention of health service or education providers, and thus the more likely it is that his or her difficulties are identified and diagnosed. As a result of both the natural history of CP and the organization of services, prevalence rates of CP ascertained during the first few years of childhood are likely to underestimate the actual rate throughout the childhood years.

Thus, in reading any account of incidence or prevalence, it is important to be aware that there are several ways in which data can be collected and reported. The most valid data are those taken from actual counts and those that are collected using systematic sampling strategies, well-defined descriptions of the conditions of interest, multiple ascertainment methods (e.g. independent confirmation of diagnosis by expert clinicians as opposed to parent report only) and a comprehensive review of all the relevant records.

What do we know about the incidence and prevalence of cerebral palsy?

Despite challenges related to diagnosing CP and deciding the age at which a definite diagnosis can be made (many people would say by age 3y), prevalence rates determined through rigorous and very large studies are remarkably stable. The information in Table 2.1 reflects data from a number of high-quality prevalence studies reported in the past 20 years. The prevalence rate for CP has been reported at about 2 to 2.5 per 1000 children in the Western world, and this figure has changed very little over the past 40 years.

Some small variation can be identified in the figures between the individual studies presented in Table 2.1. At least some of this is likely to be explained by the factors described in the sections above. For example, studies by both Kirby et al. (2011) and Surman et al. (2009a,b) included children in whom the diagnosis was made when the child was young (thus potentially including children with developmental disabilities other than CP). However, the Surman study required the diagnoses to be confirmed between the ages of 5 and 7 years. Owing to this, it is possible that the prevalence rate in the Kirby et al. study included children who *appeared* to have CP when they were young when in fact they did not have it, while these children would have been excluded from the Surman study.

Another example is the study by Krageloh-Mann et al. (1994), which reports a prevalence rate that is lower than the other studies. The focus of that study was solely on children with bilateral spastic CP. The definition for inclusion, therefore, meant that only a proportion of children with CP participated, which naturally would result in a lower prevalence.

It is also possible that the differences in prevalence figures between studies reflect, at least to an extent, a true variation in rates of CP between regions and/or populations. There is substantial evidence (e.g. Surman et al. 2009a; Wu et al. 2011) that the prevalence of CP is considerably higher among children who were born at a low birthweight. Similarly, and possibly through the same or related mechanisms, weeks of gestation (Surman et al. 2009b) and multiple births (Surman et al. 2009a) are also risk factors. Independently of the child-related factors, mothers who do not receive prenatal care and mothers' educational status have both been found to be factors relating to their child's risk of CP (Wu et al. 2011). Differences in the prevalence of CP, possibly attributable to socioeconomic differences, have been found in several studies; however, the mechanisms of this are poorly understood and it is possible that these differences are further confounded by other, yet unknown, factors (Dolk et al. 2010).

What are the patterns of cerebral palsy over time?

A number of high-quality reports and studies drawing data from large disability registers have reported decreasing rates of CP among children born over the past 20 years (e.g. Platt et al. 2007; Surman et al. 2009a,b; van Haastert et al. 2011). It is not possible to cover all these here; one paper focusing on preterm infants illustrates these points (Robertson et al. 2007).

Using sound epidemiological principles, Robertson et al. (2007) reported a 30-year perspective on the rates of CP in very preterm infants in Northern Alberta, Canada. The study used a clear definition of CP, a reliable approach to classification and rigorous methods (a prospective population-based longitudinal study with consistent follow-up supplemented with relevant contextual birth rate data). The diagnosis was confirmed for each child at the age of 3 years or older by a consistent group of expert clinicians. The study assessed changes in gestational age-specific prevalence rates of CP among extremely preterm infants born between 1973 and 2003.

Based on the excellent methodology, the findings can be considered valid and, in terms of what we have learned about CP in this high-risk population, particularly important. The investigators found that

- Overall, at age 2 years, 142 out of 1000 infant survivors of preterm birth had CP.

- The population-based survival of those born at a gestational age of 20 to 25 weeks increased from 4% in 1973 to 31% in the 3-year period 1992 to 1994 ($p<0.001$).

- The prevalence of CP per 1000 live births in those born at 20 to 25 weeks *increased* from 0 to 110 from 1973 to the years 1992 to 1994 ($p<0.001$).

- The prevalence of CP per 1000 live births in those born at 20 to 25 weeks *decreased* to 22 in the years 2001 to 2003 ($p<0.001$).

- The population-based survival of those born at a gestational age of 26 to 27 weeks increased from 23% in 1973 to between 75% and 80% in the 3-year period 1992 to 1994 ($p<0.001$).

- The prevalence of CP per 1000 live births in those born at 26 to 27 weeks increased from 15 to 155 until the years 1992 to 1994 ($p<0.001$).

- The prevalence of CP per 1000 live births in those born at 26 to 27 weeks decreased to 16 in the years 2001 to 2003 ($p<0.001$).

- For all preterm survivors born in the years 2001 to 2003, the prevalence of CP was 19 per 1000 live births.

The strengths of this study included the categorization ('stratification') of the findings by the combination of birth years and gestational age, and the contrast of patterns of survival and prevalence of CP across the whole period. The study allowed investigators to report with confidence that 'Population-based CP prevalence rates for children whose gestational age was 20 to 27 weeks and whose birthweight ranged from 500 to 1249g show steady reductions in the last decade with stable or reducing mortality, reversing trends prior to 1992–1994.'

This study clearly illustrates the point that what we know about patterns of CP has to be carefully interpreted in light of the context of the time and place in which the studies took place and taking account of trends in preterm births and the survival patterns associated with conditions such as preterm birth.

Epidemiological and clinical perspectives provide complementary information

There are essential differences between clinical assessment information and the type of data that can be obtained in epidemiological studies. Both approaches are important for understanding CP, but they serve very different purposes. This final section of the present chapter discusses the differences between clinical and epidemiological perspectives to CP, and how these can complement each other.

The essential differences between population-based data and clinical information about individuals concern (1) the degree of detail one can gather in each situation and (2) how those details can be used. In the case of a clinical assessment of an individual child with CP, we wish to have as complete a picture as possible of that person's abilities, goals and needs. This information is crucial as it allows us to individualize how we counsel that family and plan services for that child and family. However, that information is limited insofar as the specific elements of that child's and family's story, including any aetiological factors that might have been important in the genesis of CP for that child, cannot be generalized to CP in the whole population. For example, if we assess an individual child and find that the child has a recognizable pattern of brain maldevelopment and CP, we cannot assume that the brain maldevelopment is the 'cause' of the CP. Even if we had observed this in number of children, we can only hypothesize that there *may be a connection*; further, rigorous scientific *studies of causality* would then be needed to test the hypotheses.

Epidemiological information, on the other hand, enables us to look for patterns (including risk factors and outcomes) across either a representative sample or across the whole population of interest. The ultimate aim is not to understand or tailor services for an individual but to make generalizations of the whole group of children with CP and their families. Thus, for example, the identification of the very large increased risk of CP among preterm infants with a low birthweight points to the importance of a systematic follow-up of this population. This also points to the need to understand the neurobiological processes and perhaps the 'causal pathways' that predispose the less-formed brain of the preterm infant to an increased risk of being damaged by forces and 'insults' that lead to the clinical picture we call CP (Stanley et al. 2000).

Table 2.1 Prevalence of cerebral palsy in the Western world, presented in order of the most recent year of study

Authors[a]	Country of study	Year(s) of the study	Age[b] (y)	Prevalence[c] (95% CI)	Data source	Number surveyed[d]
Kirby et al. (2011)	USA	2006	2–8	3.3 (3.1–3.7)	Surveillance programme	142 338
Andersen et al. (2008)	Norway	2003–2006	4	2.1 (CI n.r.)	Survey of hospitals and rehabilitation records	178 095
Sigurdardottir et al. (2009)	Iceland	1997–2003	4–10	2.3 (1.8–3.0)	Disability register	29 137
Surman et al. (2009a)	UK	1984–2003	7	2.0 (1.9–2.6)	Disability register	688 018
Himmelmann et al. (2010)	Sweden	1999–2002	4–8	2.18 (CI n.r.)	Disability register	85 737
Dolk et al. (2010)	UK and Northern Ireland	1984–1997	5	2.2 (CI n.r.)	Disability register	1 657 569
Colver et al. (2000)	UK	1989–1993	–	2.5 (CI n.r.)	Disability register	47 691
Boyle et al. (1996)	USA	1991	3–10	2.4 (CI n.r.)	Review of a range of records related to disabilities in children	249 500[e]
Kavcic and Paret (1998)	Slovenia	1981–1990	5	3.0 (2.8–3.2)	Disability register	258 585

Study	Country	Years	Age	Prevalence rate	Source	Number of children
Pharoah et al. (1998)	UK	1984–1989	n.r.	2.1 (CI n.r.)	Disability register	789 411
Grether et al. (1992) Cummins et al. (1993)	USA	1986–1988	3	1.23 (1.1–1.4)	Disability register	155 636
Surveillance of Cerebral Palsy in Europe (2011)	Europe[f]	1980–1988	4	2.1 (2.0–2.1)	Surveillance register	2 954 326
MacGillivray and Campbell (1995)	UK	1969–1988	n.r.	2.1 (CI n.r.)	Disability register	236 920
Krageloh-Mann et al. (1994)	Germany, Sweden	1975–1986	5	1.18[g] (1.1–1.3)	Survey of health and education records	434 196
Stanley and Watson (1992)	Australia	1983–1985	5	2.2 (CI n.r.)	Disability register	68 525

[a]Full references for all studies presented within the table are found at the end of the chapter. [b]'Age' refers to the age at which a confirmed diagnosis was considered possible. [c]For consistency across studies, prevalence rates have been expressed as rates per 1000 children. [d]Number of individuals reviewed or surveyed in this particular study (the denominator). [e]Estimated number of children aged 3 to 10 years in the area in 1990. [f]Results reported in this table are based on 13 regions across France, Germany, Ireland, Italy, the Netherlands, Sweden and the UK. [g]This study included only children with bilateral spastic cerebral palsy, which is likely to explain the lower prevalence rate. CI, confidence interval; n.r., not reported.

Epidemiological and clinical perspectives provide complementary information, and drawing on both of these perspectives facilitates better planning, organization and delivery of services. An illustrative example of this is the Northern Ireland Cerebral Palsy Register (Parkes et al. 2005). Inclusion of clinical information about the severity of the children's disabilities (e.g. the numbers of children with different types of limitations in ability and activity) in the register enables service planners at local, regional and national levels to organize and deliver services on a more informed basis. Furthermore, monitoring trends over time in this type of information enables service providers to detect changes in service needs early, and thus plan ahead for challenges such as the transition to adulthood. For example, the service providers would know how many young people entering the community in the next decade would be likely to need assisted living arrangements, powered mobility aids and support in acquiring employment.

Nevertheless, there are almost always limitations to the number and quality of the clinical data that are collected in epidemiological studies. In large part this is because these data have to be decided upon prospectively, at a time when epidemiological studies are planned. The data must also be collected in standardized ways that do not easily allow for the detection and recording of specific details about individuals. As the collections must be consistent over time (to allow comparisons and monitoring of trends), it is not appropriate to change the data collection methods (e.g. to include additional clinical questions). In addition, the focus of epidemiological studies ('wide' in scope but rarely 'deep' in clinical detail) precludes collection of the amount and type of information one can gather in the clinical encounter with the individual child and the family.

One of the ways that the epidemiological and clinical approaches can be brought together concerns the issue of confirming that a child has CP as opposed to another condition. In the clinical context at the level of the individual and their family, it is important to respond to concerns identified at any age, including making decisions about relevant investigations and counselling parents to the best of our ability. In the epidemiology context at the level of the population, it is important to be certain that when we talk about CP and its associated features we really are discussing 'CP' and not other conditions. For both clinical and epidemiological purposes, continued reassessment of the child's status will enable us to evaluate changes over time and recognize both improvements and perhaps the onset of newly emerging difficulties (such as epilepsy). There may be times when there is such great change or improvement that we are left uncertain as to whether the child has 'outgrown' their CP or ever actually had CP (as opposed to developmental motor difficulties of an unspecified but perhaps temporary nature, or simply developmental variation) (see Nelson and Ellenberg 1982).

A good example of how this works well in practice is the approach adopted by the Surveillance of Cerebral Palsy in Europe group (Cans 2000; Surveillance of Cerebral Palsy Network) (see Chapter 4). Children across a large number of CP registries in Europe are 'identified' during the preschool years and entered into the registry as a possible 'case'. However, only after the age of 4 years are they formally confirmed as having or not having CP. The rationale for this process is that while impairment in motor development may be recognized at virtually any (young) age, the designation 'CP' may be unclear in many situations in the early years. As noted above, some children appear to 'outgrow' what had been labelled 'CP'. In other situations, children's emerging developmental picture may lead one to recognize any of a host of other developmental conditions. These may include conditions such as neurodegenerative disorders or global developmental slowness ('developmental retardation' or 'learning disability'[b]) that no longer 'look like' CP by the time a child is 4 years old. The Surveillance of Cerebral Palsy in Europe approach to the ascertainment of CP tries to ensure that those children who are counted and described as having CP do in fact have it and not another condition. It is in this way that the 'clinical' and 'population-based' approaches to CP are reconciled, so that one can have reasonable confidence in the conclusions and generalizations drawn from data such as these.

References

Andersen GL, Irgensb LM, Haagaasa I, Skranesc JS, Mebergd AE, Vike T (2008) Cerebral palsy in Norway: prevalence, subtypes and severity. *Eur J Paediatr Neurol* 12: 4–13.

Boyle CA, Decoufle P, Yeargin-Allsopp M (1994) Prevalence and health impact of developmental disabilities in US children. *Pediatrics* 93: 399–403.

Boyle CA, Yeargin-Allsopp M, Doernberg NS, Holmgreen P, Murphy CC, Schendel DE (1996) Prevalence of selected developmental disabilities in children 3–10 years of age: the Metropolitan Atlanta Developmental Disabilities Surveillance Program, 1991. *MMWR CDC Surveill Summs* 45: 1–14.

Bradley DM, Parsons EP, Clarke AJ (1993) Experience with screening newborns for Duchenne muscular dystrophy in Wales. *Br Med J* 306: 357–60.

Cans C (2000) Surveillance of cerebral palsy in Europe: a collaboration of cerebral palsy surveys and registers. *Dev Med Child Neurol* 42: 816–24.

Colver A, Gibson M, Hey E, Jarvis S, Mackie P, Richmond S (2000) Increasing rates of cerebral palsy across the severity spectrum in north-east England 1964–1993. *Arch Dis Child Fetal Neonatal Ed* 83: F1–12.

Cummins SK, Nelson KB, Grether JK, Velie EM (1993) Cerebral palsy in four northern California counties, births 1983 through 1985*. *J Pediatr* 123: 230–7.

Dolk H, Pattenden S, Bonellie S et al. (2010) Socio-economic inequalities in cerebral palsy prevalence in the United Kingdom: a register-based study. *Paediatr Perinat Epidemiol* 24: 149–55.

Eliasson A, Krumlinde-Sundholm L, Rösblad B et al. (2006) The Manual Ability Classification System (MACS) for children with cerebral palsy: scale development and evidence of validity and reliability. *Dev Med Child Neurol* 48: 549–59.

Grether JK, Cummins SK, Nelson KB (1992) The California Cerebral Palsy Project. *Paediatr Perinatal Epidemiol* 6: 339–51.

van Haastert IC, Groenendaal F, Uiterwaal CS et al. (2011) Decreasing incidence and severity of cerebral palsy in prematurely born children. *J Pediatr* 159: 86–91.

Himmelmann K, Hagberg G, Uvebrant P (2010) The changing panorama of cerebral palsy in Sweden. X. Prevalence and origin in the birth-year period 1999–2002. *Acta Paediatr* 99: 1337–43.

Hong T, Paneth N (2008) Maternal and infant thyroid disorders and cerebral palsy. *Semin Perinatol* 32: 438–45.

---

b   DSM-IV usage: mental retardation.

Kavcic A, Perat MV (1998) Prevalence of cerebral palsy in Slovenia: birth years 1981 to 1990. *Dev Med Child Neurol* 40: 459–63.

Kirby RS, Wingate MS, Van Naarden Braun K et al. (2011) Prevalence and functioning of children with cerebral palsy in four areas of the United States in 2006: a report from the Autism and Developmental Disabilities Monitoring Network. *Res Dev Disabil* 32: 462–9.

Krageloh-Mann I, Hagberg C, Meisner C et al. (1994) Bilateral spastic cerebral palsy – a comparative study between South-West Germany and Western Sweden. II: Epidemiology. *Dev Med Child Neurol* 36: 473–83.

Kuban KC, Allred EN, O'Shea M, Paneth N, Pagano M, Leviton A; ELGAN Study Cerebral Palsy-Algorithm Group (2008) An algorithm for identifying and classifying cerebral palsy in young children. *J Pediatr* 153: 466–72.

MacGillivray I, Campbell DM (1995) The changing pattern of cerebral palsy in Avon. *Paediatr Perinatal Epidemiol* 9: 146–55.

Mason A, Banerjee S, Eapen V, Zeitlin H, Robertson MM (1998) The prevalence of Tourette syndrome in a mainstream school population. *Dev Med Child Neurol* 40: 292–6.

Missiuna C, Smits C, Rosenbaum P, Woodside J, Law P (2001) *The prevalence of childhood disability: facts and issues*. A report prepared for the Ontario Ministry of Health and Long-term Care by *CanChild* Centre for Childhood Disability Research. Hamilton, ON: *CanChild* Centre, McMaster University.

Nelson KB, Ellenberg KH (1982) Children who 'outgrew' cerebral palsy. *Pediatrics* 69: 529–36.

Palisano R, Rosenbaum P, Walter S, Russell D, Wood E, Galuppi B (1997) Development and reliability of a system to classify gross motor function in children with cerebral palsy. *Dev Med Child Neurol* 39: 214–23.

Palisano RJ, Rosenbaum P, Bartlett D, Livingston MH (2008) Content validity of the expanded and revised Gross Motor Function Classification System. *Dev Med Child Neurol* 50: 744–50.

Parkes J, Dolk H, Hill N (2005) *Children and young people with cerebral palsy in Northern Ireland – birth years 1977–1997*. A comprehensive report from the Northern Ireland Cerebral Palsy Register. Belfast: Queen's University.

Pharoah PO, Cooke T, Johnson MA, King R, Mutch L (1998) Epidemiology of cerebral palsy in England and Scotland, 1984–9. *Arch Dis Child Fetal Neonatal Ed* 79: F21–5.

Platt MJ, Cans C, Johnson A et al. (2007) Trends in cerebral palsy among infants of very low birthweight (<1500 g) or born prematurely (<32 weeks) in 16 European centres: a database study. *Lancet* 369: 43–50.

Robertson CMT, Watt M-J, Yasui Y (2007) Changes in the prevalence of cerebral palsy for children born very prematurely within a population-based program over 30 years. *JAMA* 297: 2733–40.

Rosenbaum PL (2006) Variation and 'abnormality': recognizing the differences. Invited editorial. *J Pediatr* 149: 593–4.

Rosenbaum P, Paneth N, Leviton A, Goldstein M, Bax M (2007) Definition and classification document. In: Baxter P (ed.) *The Definition and Classification of Cerebral Palsy. Dev Med Child Neurol* 49 (Suppl 2): 8–14.

Stanley FJ, Watson L (1992) Trends in perinatal mortality and cerebral palsy in Western Australia, 1967 to 1985. *BMJ* 304: 1658–63.

Stanley FJ, Blair E, Alberman E (2000) *Cerebral Palsies: Epidemiology and Causal Pathways*. London: Mac Keith Press.

Sigurdardottir S, Thorkelsson T, Halldorsdottir M, Thorkelsson O, Vik T (2009) Trends in prevalence and characteristics of cerebral palsy among Icelandic children born 1990 to 2003. *Dev Med Child Neurol* 51: 356–63.

Surman G, Hemming K, Platt MJ et al. (2009a) Children with cerebral palsy: severity and trends over time. *Paediatr Perinat Epidemiol* 23: 513–21.

Surman G, Newdick H, King A, Davenport H, Kurinczuk JJ (2009b) *4Child Four Counties Database of Cerebral Palsy, Vision Loss and Hearing Loss in Children Annual Report*. Oxford: National Perinatal Epidemiology Unit, University of Oxford.

Surveillance of Cerebral Palsy Network. Surveillance of cerebral palsy in Europe. Available at: http://www-rheop.ujf-grenoble.fr/scpe2/site_scpe/index.php (accessed 12 January 2011).

World Health Organization (2007) *International Classification of Functioning, Disability and Health – Children and Youth Version. ICF-CY,* 1st edn. Geneva: World Health Organization.

Wu YW, Xing G, Fuentes-Afflick E, Danielson B, Smith LH, Gilbert WM (2011) Racial, ethnic, and socioeconomic disparities in the prevalence of cerebral palsy. *Pediatrics* 127: e674–e681.

Chapter 3

Aetiological considerations

Overview

We begin this chapter with a brief discussion of causal pathways and the challenges of establishing causation (an issue also discussed in Chapter 6). The majority of the text addresses what is known about causal factors in cerebral palsy (CP), organized by the timing of events, from maternal and intrauterine factors to recognized postnatal causes of brain impairment.

Distilling a summary of what is known from the vast amount of published work in this field inevitably leads to selection based on the authors' own knowledge and interests. However, because one of the first questions that parents of children with CP ask is 'Why did this happen?', it is appropriate that we summarize in this chapter the information that is available.

Before doing so, two introductory points need to be made. The first is to discuss the potential complexity of causal pathways. Take as an example a child who presents with bilateral CP and in whom magnetic resonance brain imaging demonstrates that there are neuronal migration abnormalities. We know that these radiological findings are the neuropathological basis of CP and that they are likely to have been determined during the second trimester of gestation. But why has this pathological development occurred? Possibilities include a genetically determined disorder that expresses itself in this way, a discrete antenatal event such as fetal trauma or fetal infection, or a developmental occurrence that appears to present sporadically.

Another example is that of maternal illness that leads to non-optimal fetal status, preterm birth and a requirement for neonatal intensive care, with the infant ultimately demonstrating evidence of structural impairment of the brain. This concept is important, because identifying the aetiological sequence can be a stepping stone to the provision of appropriate interventions that may lead to the prevention of CP in other children.

It is important, therefore, to consider briefly what we describe as 'levels of causation' and to recognize that there may be predisposing, precipitating, perpetuating and protective factors that combine to determine an outcome. In Chapter 6 we report how to apply rules of 'critical appraisal' to the assessment of aetiology, and in Chapter 10 we discuss the issue of causation as it relates to the challenge of assessing whether treatments 'work' in the way we hope they do. In reality, one faces the same challenge when seeking to know whether an exposure 'causes' CP as one faces when wishing to be confident that a treatment 'causes' an effect.

Establishing causality is almost always challenging. For one thing, a temporal relationship between events – one event preceding the other – can lead one to assume that there is an association between the earlier and later events, even a causal association, where possibly none exists. As discussed in Chapter 6, this concept is captured in the legal term 'post hoc ergo propter hoc' (literally 'after this, therefore because of this'). Suppose, for example, that an infant experiences perinatal difficulties, requires attention in a special care unit and is later found to have CP. In this scenario it is tempting to assume that the perinatal difficulties 'caused' the CP. However, as we discuss elsewhere in this chapter, one must ask whether the perinatal difficulties were themselves 'caused' by pre-existing difficulties that predisposed the infant to experience peri- or postnatal difficulties. These antecedent difficulties ('causes') are increasingly being recognized with modern imaging techniques that allow us to date the timing of 'insults' to neural development. In these circumstances, the observed perinatal problems (perhaps precipitated by the biological stresses associated with delivery) are an epiphenomenon – a 'marker' of other factors of which they are a result. Of course, it is also possible that perinatal problems may exacerbate the effects of a predisposing problem, but also be moderated by protective factors (e.g. effective postnatal care with modern techniques such as head cooling or pharmacological interventions) that attenuate the biological stresses to which the infant has been exposed. However, as we hope this brief discussion illustrates, making just a causal connection between earlier and later events is almost certainly overly simplistic.

The second introductory point to make is that it is not at all uncommon in our experience for the causes of CP in an individual child never to be clearly ascertained, even after comprehensive enquiries have been completed. Under these circumstances we do not dispute that there must be a cause or multiple causes; rather, our view is that in the light of current knowledge, the cause is not always known or knowable in every situation. As is discussed in Chapter 6, this can be a difficult concept to explain and can be a source of dissatisfaction and unhappiness for both parents and doctors.

It should be apparent that it is quite impossible to give a figure to the proportion of individuals with CP whose causation can be ascertained. Based upon clinical experience, it may well be that informed guesswork as to probable causes can be made for around 80% of children with CP. By contrast, when we attempt to discover the precise mechanisms of causation, the proportion for which this can be done probably falls to less than 20%.

When considering aetiology, it is therefore probably most useful to examine this idea within a number of possible time epochs. These are preconceptual, intrauterine (with this grouping being divided into approximately the first half and then the second half of gestation), perinatal including intrapartum, and postnatal.

In Chapter 1, we indicated that CP can be regarded as a model for developmental neurodisability. When considering aetiology, CP can again be regarded as a model. Therefore, similar considerations would apply if other developmental disabilities such as epilepsy, cognitive impairment or autistic spectrum disorder were being evaluated.

The development and implementation into practice of magnetic resonance brain imaging has been a key development in making it possible to identify the link between the identification of the clinical features of CP and the identification of the presence of structural brain abnormalities. Before the advent of brain imaging, assumptions were made from clinically observing groups of children and correlating the findings with their antecedent circumstances. The state of knowledge 20 years ago was summarized by Ellenberg and Nelson (1988), who stated that CP is often associated with a series of suboptimal conditions occurring between conception and the perinatal period rather than with a single insult. As a consequence of what has been learned from brain imaging, much more information is now available on the patterns of brain injury. This information is well illustrated by Bax et al. (2006).

Against this background, events in the various time epochs identified above can now be considered.

Preconceptual events

Identified genetic causes
Among children who fulfil the diagnostic criteria for CP, there are very few known genetic 'causes'. By contrast, many genetically determined disorders that present with symmetrical spasticity, for example hereditary spastic paraplegia, or dystonia with or without athetosis, such as Lesch–Nyhan syndrome or glutaric aciduria type I, are ultimately progressive. There are, however, a number of case reports of children with bilateral spastic CP who have two or more siblings without CP. The literature on this subject was summarized as long ago as 1992 (Hughes and Newton 1992). McHale et al. (1999) have taken this a step further and identified a gene on chromosome 2q24–25 that is linked with symmetrical spastic CP.

The clinical message is that there is a need for a critical consideration of aetiology in all children with CP, because there is a low threshold for referral for a clinical genetics opinion if a probable cause is not readily ascertainable. There are no published data that indicate what proportion of children with CP are referred for genetic advice as this is determined by both local practice and available services.

Predisposing and Predictive Prenatal Factors
Many factors may act in an indirect or a more specific way and can be regarded as risk factors. They may include adverse socioeconomic status, as is the case for learning disabilities (DSM-IV usage: mental retardation) (Shevell et al. 2000), smoking and alcohol, as well as specific maternal health problems such as diabetes, maternal rhesus isoimmunization acquired at the time of a previous pregnancy and individual thrombophilic conditions such as maternal anti-phospholipid syndrome (for which genetic underpinnings are increasingly being recognized). None is a direct cause of CP, but each may turn out to be part of a causal chain that will require full evaluation in individual cases.

Early antenatal factors
What is surprising in clinical neonatology and paediatric practice is how infrequently a specific early antenatal cause for CP is identified. There are no published data that quantify this, but we have the clinical impression that antenatal causes are assumed for no more than around 5% of children with CP . These causes include chromosomal abnormalities that occur in association with early cell division after fertilization, although more often these will cause overall developmental delay rather than CP. They also include congenital infections, of which the best recognized are rubella and cytomegalovirus. The spectrum of impairment under these circumstances almost always includes a host of neurodevelopmental problems in addition to those of motor function.

Other 'causes' of CP include early cerebral malformation syndromes where, as has been indicated, the question must inevitably arise as to what has been the precursor for this abnormal development. The range of malformations includes anencephaly at its most severe, disorders of neuronal proliferation such as hemimegalencephaly, disorders of neuronal migration including lissencephaly and heterotopias, and disorders of neuronal organization including schizencephaly and polymicrogyria. It should be made clear that within this grouping the disorders of organization occur late in the second trimester, and they are included here for convenience.

The point also needs to be made that while some of the more severe cerebral malformations are lethal either during gestation or during the course of early childhood, those that are responsible for CP do not appear to have a major adverse effect on fetal viability in utero. The majority of children affected by cerebral malformation syndromes are born at term. It is only when evidence of developmental delay or CP becomes apparent and the children are investigated that the diagnosis is made. In clinical practice this is usually within the first year of life, but this does depend on the level of functional impairment that brings the child to attention and the threshold for undertaking investigations being suitably low.

The diagnosis of cerebral malformation is made after postnatal magnetic resonance brain imaging if the resulting clinical abnormalities are those of CP, which is usually but not invariably bilateral, together in most cases with overall developmental retardation and epilepsy.

Leaving aside these identifiable aetiologies, what is disappointing to parents and clinicians alike is that full investigations, including magnetic resonance brain imaging, are so often normal or unhelpfully non-specific. It follows that, particularly in the first half of gestation, there is currently a paucity of identified and identifiable causes of brain damage. In clinical practice, the assumption is therefore often made that a child's problems have arisen at a subtle cellular or neurochemical level. While this may be correct, not only is it intellectually unsatisfying but also, more importantly, it does not provide helpful or useful information to parents, for example about recurrence risk.

Later antenatal factors

It is not surprising, given the more advanced fetal maturation that has occurred, that more is known about the causes and associations of CP that derive from the second half of gestation. As has been indicated above, these can include disorders of neuronal proliferation, and it is of interest that although most of these are developmental brain abnormalities, some can be acquired disorders. They have been recognized, for example, as a consequence of fetal cerebrovascular disorders and after fetal injuries such as may be sustained in a road traffic accident involving the mother (Hayes et al. 2007).

There are no particular correlations between the patterns of CP and the underlying brain malformation other than that the general point can be made that the more diffuse and extensive the brain abnormality, the more severe are the features of CP and other developmental manifestations seen in the affected child.

Periventricular leukomalacia

Fetal viability has been achieved at around 24 weeks of gestation, and the common link between brain-damaging processes that occur at 24 to 34 weeks of gestation is preterm birth.

Being born preterm does not cause brain damage but is a risk factor. Whether the risks are translated into damage depends upon the cause(s) of the preterm birth, on the perinatal factors that apply in individual circumstances, on how the fetus adapts to extrauterine life and on the quality of neonatal care. Brain vulnerability between 26 and 34 weeks of gestational age is seen particularly in the cerebral hemispheric white matter close to the lateral ventricles, and there is also a risk of germinal matrix haemorrhage into the lateral ventricles early in postnatal life.

So far as the cerebral hemispheric white matter is concerned, the result of the damaging process is often described as periventricular leukomalacia (PVL). It is necessary to make clear, however, that this is a non-specific term describing the location (around the ventricles) of softened white matter (leukomalacia) and does not imply either a specific cause or a specific pathology.

What is known, however, is that the periventricular white matter is a vulnerable area of the brain at this gestational age and its structure and function can be adversely affected by a variety of causative pathologies. They include ischaemia deriving from hypoxia or other circulatory disturbance, and can occur either before, during the course of or after preterm birth. Another recognized major risk factor is maternal chorioamnionitis, which can occur after premature rupture of the membranes with resulting ascending maternal infection. Under those circumstances, maternal cytokines (chemicals mobilized to fight infection) are believed to have an adverse effect on the oligodendroglia (the cells that are responsible for white matter production).

After birth, overventilation leading to documented hypocarbia in the neonate is also recognized as a causal factor for periventricular white matter damage. Other causes and interrelationships are also described, and the subject has been reviewed in detail by Volpe (2001).

Whenever the events that determine the development of PVL occur, the evolution of brain changes tends to be seen postnatally and can be followed by serial imaging using ultrasound, computed tomography or magnetic resonance brain scanning. There is a close but not invariable association between the recognition on imaging of PVL and the development of CP. The characteristic form of CP that is seen under these circumstances has historically been described as diplegia, a term about which there is controversy, as discussed in Chapter 4.

The clinical hallmark of this form of CP is motor developmental delay that is associated with spastic hypertonus that principally affects the lower limbs. However, the spectrum of impairment in children who are labelled as diplegic can be very wide indeed (see Gorter et al. 2004) and this has led to a recommendation that the term diplegia should be abandoned, as is discussed in Chapter 4. The spectrum of disability that is seen in diplegic CP is also detailed in Chapter 4.

In general, the severity of the motor disorder and of the associated impairments that are present in diplegic CP corresponds well with the extent of demonstrated brain damage.

Intraventricular haemorrhage

Infants who are born preterm are at risk of sustaining germinal matrix haemorrhage within the lateral ventricles; the greater the degree of prematurity, the more likely it is that bleeding will occur. They are also at risk of periventricular venous infarction. This can cause brain damage as a consequence of hydrocephalus with resulting raised intracranial pressure (termed posthaemorrhagic hydrocephalus) and as a consequence of the haemorrhagic infarction extending into the brain parenchyma. Under these circumstances the clinical sequelae can include motor developmental delay with hypotonia or more severe forms of CP. Intraventricular haemorrhage can also occur concurrently with PVL; under those circumstances, the likelihood is that there will be more functionally severe motor disability.

Cerebral palsy of perinatal origin in term-born infants

Hypoxic–ischaemic injury

Time has moved on considerably since all forms of CP were considered to be due to brain damage at birth. The swings of the pendulum that have been seen over our professional lifetimes have been influenced by critical inquiry, an increased understanding of pathogenetic mechanisms, work derived from animal studies and the influence of litigation. As with the time epochs from which CP derives, the advent and widespread use of magnetic resonance brain imaging has been of fundamental importance in contributing to an understanding of the nature and timing of brain development and the brain-damaging processes that may occur.

There now appears to be a consensus that there are two largely, albeit not wholly, discrete patterns of brain injury that can occur perinatally. In the first, the final common pathway is perfusion failure affecting the cerebral hemispheres. This is also called 'hypoxic–ischaemic brain injury', to which the descriptive phrase 'prolonged partial hypoxia' is often added.

What has been established is that either in the last few days or weeks of gestation or during the course of labour and delivery, effective brain circulation is compromised. The fetus may have an enhanced vulnerability to this development as a consequence of maternal health issues including pre-eclampsia or other factors that have caused the fetus to fail to thrive satisfactorily in utero.

It is sometimes the case that biophysical parameters are of assistance in recognizing this development, and under those circumstances it may be appropriate for delivery to be expedited. A compromise of effective fetal cerebral circulation can also occur in labour and may be marked by cardiotocographic changes.

Rules of thumb suggest that a fetus can cope with at least an hour of prolonged partial hypoxia in labour before brain damage due to perfusion failure begins. However, the science that forms the basis of this argument is unclear, although the work of Myers (1975) and Pasternak (2003) is often cited.

The pattern of brain damage that occurs when there is cerebral perfusion failure is often described as 'watershed' cerebral hemispheric infarction. This implies that infarction occurs in the areas between the territories of the major cerebral arteries, that is between the territory of the middle and anterior cerebral artery and the middle and posterior cerebral artery, and this pattern is demonstrable on magnetic resonance brain imaging.

When children sustain brain damage in this way during the course of labour, it is usually expected that at the time of birth there will be a degree of acidosis and cardio-respiratory depression followed by the development of a neonatal encephalopathy with seizures. However, the extent of both the cardiorespiratory depression and the encephalopathy can be very variable. Affected children then go on to demonstrate the clinical picture of widespread impairment of neurological function. Commonly there is bilateral spastic CP together with evidence of overall developmental retardation. Often, too, there is microcephaly, visual impairment of brain origin and epilepsy. The clinical vignette, AA, described in Chapter 1 is characteristic of this grouping.

Another hypoxic–ischaemic causation pathway that can occur at term is that of brain damage that follows a short period of acute and profound hypoxia. Under these circumstances, damage occurs to those regions of the term brain that have a high degree of metabolic activity. Typically these are the deep grey matter structures of the thalami, lentiform nuclei and globus pallidus. The pre- and postcentral gyri of the cerebral hemispheres with their underlying white matter are also vulnerable, as are the hippocampal regions of the temporal lobes.

The causes of acute fetal compromise at term include placental abruption and events in labour such as cord prolapse and compression, uterine rupture and shoulder dystocia. The research evidence suggesting that the otherwise healthy term fetus can only survive for a period of around 10 minutes of acute and profound hypoxia before brain damage begins is rather better than is the case in prolonged partial hypoxia (Rennie and Rosenbloom 2011).

After 10 minutes, brain damage begins and appears to increase very rapidly, so that if the total period of acute and profound hypoxia exceeds 25 to 30 minutes then the fetus is likely to die or be very profoundly damaged. Infants damaged in this way usually show a very severe degree of cardiorespiratory depression at the time of birth. This is usually accompanied by a severe degree of acidosis. They usually then go on to develop a neonatal encephalopathy with seizures, although in some cases this can be subtle (Rosenbloom 1994). Affected children later demonstrate features of what is best described as a dyskinetic or dystonic bilateral CP due to extrapyramidal motor dysfunction, together with lower limb spasticity as a consequence of involvement of the motor cortex. Often there is some preservation of cognitive abilities, at least relative to the severe involvement of motor function. Brain imaging under these circumstances characteristically demonstrates signal change in the basal ganglia and in the pre- and postcentral gyri of the cerebral hemispheres.

Perinatal stroke
A neuropathology that is seen particularly in term infants and that is a cause of CP is usually described as perinatal stroke. The subject has been well reviewed by Lynch et al. (2002).

Technically, occlusion of a major cerebral blood vessel, most frequently the left middle cerebral artery, occurs either as a consequence of embolism from a remote site (thought to be the placenta when the stroke occurs antenatally) or by thrombosis in situ. It is thought that this might occur if there is an inherent thrombophilic condition affecting the fetus or newborn infant.

When this episode occurs antenatally it is clinically silent, and the infant is usually healthy in the newborn period. During the course of the first year, however, clinical evidence of a hemiplegia evolves, as is detailed in the case of child BB described in Chapter 1. Perinatal stroke can also occur in the neonatal period. Under those circumstances, it is sometimes possible to identify the embolic or thrombotic source. The newborn infant is likely to be encephalopathic (i.e. show symptoms and signs of acute neurological distress), although the degree of accompanying seizure disturbance can be mild.

Controversy exists about whether perinatal stroke occurs in labour as a consequence of adverse factors that operate in the labour. Information is not available as to the precise mechanisms that are operative under this circumstance, although the suggestion has been made that emboli deriving from the fetal side of the placenta can be dislodged in association with uterine contractions.

The clinical correlate of perinatal stroke is usually a hemiplegia, that is unilateral CP, as is discussed further in Chapter 4. There is also an increased risk of cognitive impairment, epilepsy and behavioural disturbance. Confirmation of the existence and extent of the presence of focal cerebral infarction is derived from brain imaging.

Other perinatal causes

Other perinatal causes include neonatal hyperbilirubinaemia producing kernicterus. The resulting clinical picture usually features an extrapyramidal syndrome and hearing loss together, usually with cognitive impairment and often also epilepsy. Magnetic resonance brain imaging may show an abnormal signal in the globus pallidus.

Symptomatic neonatal hypoglycaemia with seizures also has the potential to cause brain damage with features of CP. However, the more obvious features seen clinically are cognitive and visual impairment and epilepsy. Other causes include birth trauma and neonatal infection; the clinical history is usually evident in these circumstances.

Postnatal causes

As has already been indicated, it is not possible to provide an agreed age at which it is universally accepted that 'CP' can be caused by postnatal brain impairment, although many clinicians regard the age of 2 years as being a useful working time. Again, and as has already been made clear (see Chapter 1), many of the clinical, service delivery and family impact issues that relate to CP are also seen in brain injury acquired later in childhood and need to be addressed in the same ways.

There have been a few studies looking systematically at postnatal CP. One study is that of Pharoah et al. (1989). Bacterial infection, particularly meningitis, other inflammatory disorders and trauma, both accidental and non-accidental, are most widely represented as possible causes. Because of the availability of modern investigational techniques, it is now exceptional for a cause or causal chain not to be identifiable in children who develop their CP postnatally. It is also important to remember that in many parts of the world cerebral malaria and other infectious diseases are common causes of postnatally acquired CP (Levin 2006).

Some diagnostic care is required, however, in distinguishing conditions that may be inherently progressive, such as Rett syndrome, from conditions that have caused non-progressive brain impairment. This is an illustration of an issue discussed in Chapter 2 regarding the epidemiology of CP.

In summary, as was indicated at the beginning of this chapter, it is impossible to provide definitive estimates of the proportions of children with CP whose causation can be ascribed to these various time epochs. Against this background, and probably at least in part as a reaction to both historical beliefs and clinical negligence litigation that have suggested that adverse birth circumstances are the most common cause of CP, there has been a reaction that has tended to minimize a link between perinatal adversity and CP. This is exemplified by MacLennan (1999), who has suggested that particularly rigorous criteria need to be satisfied before such a link can be accepted. de Vries and Cowan (2009) have detailed a more balanced view.

It is our perspective that when similar causation criteria based on best available evidence are applied to all of the time epochs detailed in this chapter, less than 10% of cases of CP are determined before conception, that about the same proportion have their origin in the first half of gestation, that around 20% will derive from the second half of gestation (including the sequelae to preterm birth), that around 20% will derive from perinatal adversity at around term and less than 10% will be determined after the immediate neonatal period. The remainder (rather more than 30%) have unidentifiable aetiologies on the basis of current knowledge. It should be emphasized that this is the authors' personal view based on their experience in this field. Studies that could confirm or refute this cannot be undertaken retrospectively as relevant comprehensive data are not available.

References

Bax M, Tydeman C, Flodmark O (2006) Clinical and MRI correlates of cerebral palsy: the European Cerebral Palsy Study. *JAMA* 296: 1602–8.

Gorter JW, Rosenbaum PL, Hanna SE et al. (2004) Limb distribution, type of motor disorder and functional classification of cerebral palsy: how do they relate? *Dev Med Child Neurol* 46: 461–7.

Ellenberg JH, Nelson KB (1988) Cluster of perinatal events identifying infants at high risk for death and disability. *J Pediatr* 113: 546–52.

Hayes B, Ryan S, Stephenson JB, King MD (2007) Cerebral palsy after maternal trauma in pregnancy. *Dev Med Child Neurol* 49: 700–6.

Hughes I, Newton R (1992) Genetic aspects of cerebral palsy. *Dev Med Child Neurol* 34: 80–6.

Levin K (2006) 'I am what I am because of who we all are': international perspectives on rehabilitation: South Africa. *Pediatr Rehabil* 9: 285–92.

Lynch JK, Hirtz DG, DeVeber G, Nelson KB (2002) Report of the National Institute of Neurological Disorders and Stroke Workshop on Perinatal and Childhood Stroke. *Pediatrics* 109: 116–23.

McHale DP, Mitchell S, Bundey S et al. (1999) A gene for autosomal recessive symmetrical spastic cerebral palsy maps to chromosome Zq 24–25. *Am J Hum Genet* 64: 526–32.

MacLennan A (1999) A template for defining a causal relation between acute intrapartum events and cerebral palsy: international consensus statement. *BMJ* 319: 1054–9.

Myers RE (1975) Two patterns of brain damage and their conditions of occurrence. *Am J Obstet Gynecol* 112: 246.

Pasternak JF (2003) Hypoxic ischemic brain damage in the term infant. *Pediatr Clin North Am* 40: 1061–72.

Pharoah PO, Cooke T, Rosenbloom L (1989) Acquired cerebral palsy. *Arch Dis Child* 64: 1013–16.

Rennie J, Rosenbloom L (2011) 'How long do we have to get the baby out?' A review of the effects of acute and profound intrapartum hypoxia and ischaemia. *The Obstetrician and Gynaecologist* 13: 169–74.

Rosenbloom L (1994) Dyskinetic cerebral palsy and birth asphyxia. *Dev Med Child Neurol* 36: 285–9.

Shevell ML, Majnemer A, Rosenbaum P, Abrahamowicz M (2000) Etiologic yield of single domain developmental delay: a prospective study. *J Pediatr* 137: 633–7.

Volpe JJ (2001) Neurobiology of periventricular leukomalacia in the premature infant. *Pediatr Res* 50: 553–62.

de Vries LS, Cowan FM (2009) Evolving understanding of hypoxic-ischaemic encephalopathy in the term infant. *Semin Pediatr Neurol* 16: 216–25.

Chapter 4

How is cerebral palsy categorized, why is this done and what are the potential pitfalls?

Overview

In this chapter we make a number of recommendations about the classification of cerebral palsy (CP). In particular, we argue that we should move beyond our traditional reliance on classic descriptions of the body distribution of CP being hemiplegia, diplegia and quadriplegia; of the motor impairments being spastic, dystonic or ataxic; and of the functional limitations being called mild, moderate or severe. We propose instead that validated classification systems, designed specifically for use with people with CP, be applied consistently.

These ideas are likely to be unattractive to some clinicians. We believe that traditional terminology should be recognized to be shorthand. In the interest of clarity and communication, we hope that people will correlate these shorthand descriptions with the classifications we are recommending. There is no doubt that the universal application of consistent standard and meaningful language and terminology will enhance communication among professionals and, equally importantly, help parents and families to know what we all mean by the words and phrases we use.

Introduction to classification

The classification of CP has traditionally addressed several clinical features of the condition, thus resulting in a number of terms that are widely used. As described below, each of these ideas seems, on the surface, to be both clinically understandable and useful for differentiating individuals on the basis of these features. Unfortunately, as we shall note, what makes conceptual sense may be rather more challenging to realize in practice. However, before addressing that issue, some brief general comments about terminology are required in order to help people find their way through a host of terms that often mean the same things but are said differently and, as we will suggest, are less precise than we usually recognize.

In medicine, people have traditionally used a mix of words derived from Latin and Greek to describe things. For CP we use both languages somewhat interchangeably, for example talking about four-limb involvement as 'quadriplegia' (Latin) or 'tetraplegia' (Greek). We speak of 'palsy', which Wikipedia refers to as 'paralysis of a body part often accompanied by loss of feeling and uncontrolled body movements such as shaking' (http://en.wikipedia.org/wiki/Somatosensory_system), but we also use the suffix 'plegia', derived from Greek, which means much the same thing.

As an illustration of the looseness of the terminology, the 'palsy' of CP usually does not lead to loss of feeling, and only some forms of CP are accompanied by 'uncontrolled body movements such as shaking'. It is therefore not surprising that both parents and service providers are often confused by the words used to describe their children. This confusion not only can create anxiety for parents when they hear people describe their children using different words for the same phenomena, but also may create a sense that we are being precise and very specific when such precision does not really exist.

Another notion that is important to recognize when discussing classification is that this process is in fact an aspect of measurement. It is therefore important to consider whether any classification system 'works' as a measurement system ought to do. Is the system 'reliable' – which is to say, do different individuals who use it make similar categorizations when classifying the same person, and does an individual classify the same person the same way from one time to another when things have not changed? It is equally important to know whether the classification system is 'valid' – that is, whether it is meaningful in some way or other that helps either the people doing the classifying or the people being classified.

A further issue with respect to classification is that it assumes that the presenting clinical features are stable. As has already been indicated in Chapter 1, CP is an evolving disorder and the clinical presentations of young infants can be very different from those that are seen as the children become older. It might therefore be reasonable to argue that a minimum age should be achieved before classification for epidemiological purposes can be confirmed. As discussed in Chapter 1, this is consistent with the approach used by the Surveillance of Cerebral Palsy in Europe (SCPE) group, according to which confirmation of the diagnosis of CP is not made until children are aged 4 years. Figure 4.1, reproduced from the SCPE, presents the clinical decision-making algorithm used to decide whether a child fits the clinical diagnosis of 'CP' for epidemiological purposes. The downside of this idea is that there is a small but appreciable mortality of severely affected children in the first 2 years of life, and it is important that this group be recognized in population and other epidemiological studies.

In discussing classification, it is important to record that various epidemiological studies of CP have used a variety of categorizations. Some of these have been determined

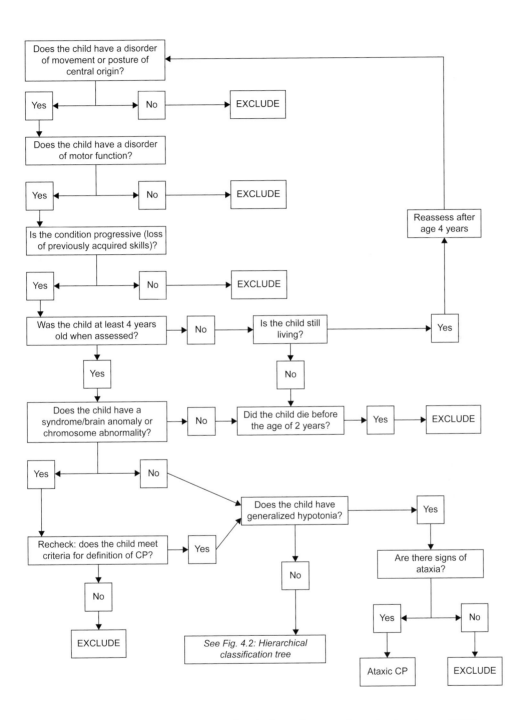

Figure 4.1 Decision tree for inclusion/exclusion of cases of cerebral palsy on SCPE register. Published with permission from Cans et al. (2000).

by researchers, some of whom have merely extracted details from clinical records. To the best of our knowledge, none of the CP epidemiology studies other than that of the SCPE have re-evaluated their populations to see if they were appropriately categorized. The differences in categorization make for difficulties in comparing various epidemiological studies.

A final introductory point is that diagnosing, classifying and categorizing individual children with CP should be based on detailed and appropriate evaluations, including an informed neurological examination. In addition, some people (Russman and Ashwal 2004) believe that, wherever possible, this should be complemented by appropriate neuroradiological information derived from magnetic resonance brain imaging.

However, given that magnetic resonance brain imaging is far from universally available, it could be argued that data obtained by imaging studies should be used to add to the detail when talking about individual children with CP, that is, imaging should be regarded as a clinical rather than a specific classification or categorization tool. Nevertheless, the European study by Bax et al. (2006) does correlate clinical 'syndromes' with imaging, and we probably need to recognize and accept this as one reasonable way of using categorization. This example illustrates that 'clinical–radiological' correlations can be helpful in advancing the field by identifying and characterizing underlying structural brain 'damage'; being able to link clinical observations to underlying structural brain findings enhances our overall understanding of CP (as discussed in Chapter 3).

Topography

The first and most obvious classification of CP concerns what parts of the body are affected by the disorder and to what extent. Some people call this the 'topography' of the condition. We speak of 'hemiplegia' or 'hemiparesis' to mean that 'half' the body (one side) is affected while the other 'half' is not. This is clinically rather similar to what one sees in an adult after a stroke, and may in fact be the equivalent of a stroke that has affected a fetus or very young child. Of course, as discussed in Chapter 2, it is important to recognize that the time in life when a stroke occurs is very significant with respect to whether the person who has the stroke is acquiring skills (as infants are expected to do over the course of their development) or is recovering them (through 'rehabilitation', as adults try to do in order to return to their previous levels of function).

One challenge with the 'hemi' designations concerns whether the 'non-hemi' side of the body is in fact fully capable (what people often call 'normal') or is simply less obviously impaired than the more involved side (Steenbergen and Meulenbroek 2006). This issue is important for at least two reasons.

First, it must be obvious that when a biological 'insult' has caused a brain impairment leading to the hemisyndrome, it may have created disturbances elsewhere in the brain, possibly resulting in additional functional limitations on the apparently 'normal' side of the body. As service providers, we may too easily focus on the obvious impairments and miss what may be more subtle signs of functional difficulties elsewhere. The corollary of this observation is the possibility that we might ascribe functional difficulties observed with the non-hemi (often inappropriately labelled the 'good') side of the body to behavioural issues such as a child acting up because they have a disability or are depressed about their CP. It therefore behoves us as service providers to be careful, systematic and attentive in assessing all aspects of the person's functional abilities and challenges. We must not be distracted by focusing only on the obvious difficulties, and in the process fail to observe the whole person carefully.

Another topographical descriptive term is 'diplegia' – classically used to mean that the person's legs are more 'involved' than the upper extremities. Here, as elsewhere, this seems an obvious distinction – until one tries to make it work in practice, at which point the challenges become apparent. A brief discussion of the term will illustrate the way that concepts and clinical reality may not align.

To many clinicians, diplegia is an entity that is seen in some children who have been born significantly preterm, who may or may not have been unwell in the neonatal period, and who present with CP which is manifest by lower limb spasticity together with at least relative preservation of the upper limbs and cognitive functioning. In individual children, it is appropriate to describe their clinical presentation and functional status in detail. When using this clinical label, it is usual to anticipate that the neuropathological and neuroradiological correlates will be those of periventricular leukomalacia (PVL).

The difficulties with applying the label 'diplegia' are, however, significant. At a clinical level, it is recognized that this pattern of CP can be seen in children born at term, and that there are no hard and fast criteria that can be applied with respect to how much upper limb function has to be preserved. In addition, it is known radiologically that some children with 'diplegic' CP do not have PVL.

In the extreme and very clear situation in which a person demonstrates obvious difficulties in standing and in gait but has excellent upper extremity function, 'diplegia' is easy to see and categorize. However, in the absence of valid ways to describe and compare the function of upper extremities against lower, how do we make the distinction between 'better' upper limb function and 'worse' lower extremity function? In other words, where does 'diplegia' end and 'quadriplegia' begin? There appear to be no clear answers to this important question.

Colver and Sethumadhavan (2003) addressed these issues and argued against the retention of the term diplegia principally on the grounds that there is no consistency among clinicians on what it comprises. By contrast, some clinicians have recommended its retention given its historical place within the literature on CP and because the 'typical' case is readily recognized.

We accept that clinicians will continue to use the term diplegia. However, we would prefer that it be used in parallel with a fuller description of such individuals as having 'bilateral CP', which is usually (but not invariably) spastic. We also expect there to be some detail of the topographical distribution, an indication of Gross Motor Function Classification System (GMFCS) and Manual Ability Classification System (MACS) levels and information, if it is known, of any brain imaging abnormalities.

Turning to four-limb involvement (what Dr Eugene Bleck [1987] refers to more accurately as 'total body involvement'), professionals often unwittingly mix topography with 'severity'. In people with quadriplegia whose overall functional abilities are significantly limited, this designation is, again, easy to recognize. However, when someone with diplegia has 'some' upper limb impairment, how 'severe' does the overall picture need to be before 'diplegia' is called 'quadriplegia'? Here as elsewhere there are no sound and valid ways to make these distinctions.

The SCPE group has worked to simplify this question (Cans 2000). They have created very useful simple algorithms to enable people to 'place' a child into one of a relatively small group of mutually exclusive and collectively exhaustive functional and motor disorder categories (Fig. 4.2). With respect to the topographical distinctions described earlier in this chapter, they simply refer to unilateral and bilateral CP. Of course, as we have argued in this chapter, one still needs to be certain, at the clinical level, that the unilateral distribution clearly does affect only one side of the body.

Motor function impairment

After the body distribution of the CP has been considered, a second category of descriptors is often used to refer to the characteristics of motor function. Terms used include 'spastic', 'athetotic' (or 'choreoathetotic'), 'dystonic', 'hypotonic', 'ataxic' and of course 'mixed' CP. Once again we prefer the SCPE group's approach, in which they have created a simplified and clinically sensible categorization and definition of these terms (see Table 4.1) in which the functional descriptions are clearly laid out. These are discussed further in Chapter 9. Note should also be made of the excellent work done by Sanger et al. (2003, 2010) to describe various types of movement disorders in children, including of course motor challenges, seen in people with CP.

It will be understood that children with the spastic forms of CP primarily have corticospinal tract (pyramidal tract) dysfunction. Those with the dyskinetic forms of CP primarily have extrapyramidal motor dysfunction.

Degree of impairment

How has the 'severity' of CP been described? Classically we have used words such as 'mild', 'moderate' and 'severe' to categorize motor (and other) functional aspects of the condition. Sadly, these words have never been clearly defined so that people know what they mean. There is no evidence that different people use these terms reliably (consistently), or even whether we are consistent with ourselves over time when classifying the same person. Furthermore, these words imply judgements rather than descriptions of function. The words are relative to one another: 'mild' can easily

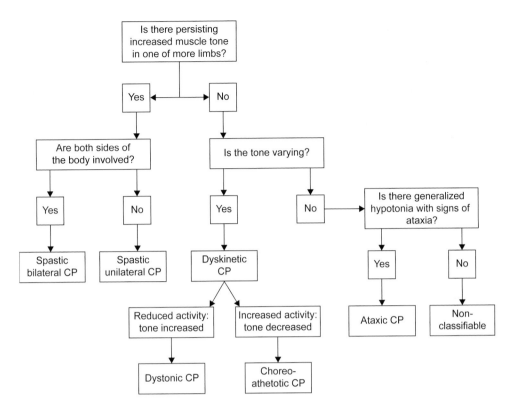

Figure 4.2 Hierarchical classification tree of cerebral palsy (CP) subtypes. Published with permission from Cans et al. (2000).

be taken to mean 'it could be worse', and 'severe' suggests a sense of hopelessness. In themselves, these descriptors convey absolutely nothing about function.

In the 1990s, the GMFCS was created, and was shown to be valid, reliable and stable over time (Palisano et al. 1997, 2006, 2008; Wood and Rosenbaum 2000; McCormick et al. 2007). The GMFCS consists of five 'levels' that describe gross motor function in several age bands (to accommodate children's natural development over time). This is simply a pattern recognition system with which the person doing the classifying matches a child's current function to the closest verbal 'picture' in the GMFCS. The functional abilities may be observed or described – this is not a test or assessment and requires no equipment or special skills. The GMFCS has been translated into many languages and is now used all over the world (Morris 2008). It has been expanded from the original 0- to 12-year descriptors to include a 12- to 18-year age band (Palisano et al. 2008). The 'Expanded and Revised' GMFCS is available for free on the Internet at http://www.canchild.ca/en/measures/gmfcs_expanded_revised.asp and is also presented in Appendix I.

Table 4.1 Definitions adopted for European classification of cerebral palsy (CP). Published with permission from Cans et al. (2000)

Spastic CP is characterized by at least two of

    Abnormal pattern of posture and/or movement

    Increased tone (not necessarily constant)

    Pathological reflexes (increased reflexes: hyperreflexia and/or pyramidal signs, e.g. Babinski response)

Spastic CP may be either bilateral or unilateral

Spastic bilateral CP is diagnosed if

    Limbs on both sides of the body are involved

Spastic unilateral CP is diagnosed if

    Limbs on one side of the body are involved

Ataxic CP is characterized by both

    Abnormal pattern of posture and/or movement

    Loss of orderly muscular coordination so that movements are performed with abnormal force, rhythm and accuracy

Dyskinetic CP is dominated by both

    Abnormal pattern of posture and/or movement

    Involuntary, uncontrolled, recurring, occasionally stereotyped movements

Dyskinetic CP may be either dystonic or choreoathetotic

    Dystonic CP is dominated by both:

        Hypokinesia (reduced activity, i.e. stiff movement)

        Hypertonia (tone usually increased)

    Choreoathetotic CP is dominated by both:

        Hyperkinesia (increased activity, i.e. stormy movement)

        Hypotonia (tone usually decreased)

It is also reasonable to make the point that of the three types of classification described here (topographical, motor 'type' and GMFCS), only the GMFCS has been developed and studied specifically as a classification tool with solid evidence of reliability and validity.

An analogue of the GMFCS has been developed to classify manual abilities (Eliasson et al. 2006). Both the GMFCS and the MACS (available at www.macs.nu; see Appendix II) categorize 'usual function' and provide verbal descriptors that can be reported reliably by parents as well as service providers (Morris et al. 2006). Both systems may also be useful as a guide to functional needs and are potentially helpful in planning interventions for individual children and young people. This is illustrated conceptually by Heinen and his colleagues (2009), who have proposed graphically how in future one may be able to take account of a child's age and GMFCS level to consider the kinds of therapies and services that might be appropriate based on these two key determinants of function.

In addition, a Communication Function Classification System (CFCS) has been created, modelled on the GMFCS and MACS (Hidecker et al. 2011). Building on the lessons learned from earlier classification developments (Rosenbaum et al. 2008), the CFCS has been developed with the input of parents and persons with CP as well as a wide range of service providers from several countries. It is available at http://cfcs.us (see Appendix III).

The topographic and motor impairment categorizations described in the first section of this chapter are often used to imply the functional status of a person with CP. At least with respect to gross motor function, people easily assume that individuals with hemisyndromes are more functional than those with diplegia, and that people with quadriplegia are least functional – and there is more than a grain of truth to that generalization. However, when the opportunity arose to explore the relationship between GMFCS levels and the classic descriptions of CP (Gorter et al. 2004) with a large, randomly selected sample of children and young people with CP, it quickly became apparent that neither the topographical nor the motor impairment categorizations aligned as closely to the GMFCS levels as had been assumed (Figs. 4.3 and 4.4).

For example, although most ($n=86$; 88%) of the 98 children and young people in the study with hemisyndromes were functioning at GMFCS level I (the best level of function), the others were classified in levels II–IV. The 217 children with diplegia were spread very widely across levels I–IV; the 263 children described as having quadriplegia were found predominantly in GMFCS levels IV and V, but a substantial proportion (23%) were functioning at levels I and II. The functional performance of children was equally variable across the several types of motor impairment described in this population.

Assessing function
As has been indicated, the classification of CP in individual children needs to be derived from clinical assessment. Within that context (discussed more fully in Chapter 12), one of the established measures for evaluating gross motor function in people with CP is the Gross Motor Function Measure (GMFM) (Russell et al. 2002). This is a purpose-designed valid and reliable descriptive and change-detecting ('evaluative') measure used

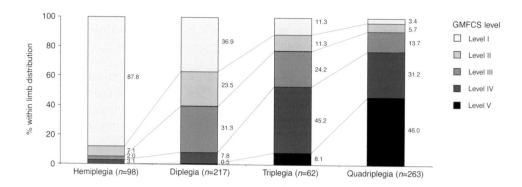

Figure 4.3 'Limb distribution' by Gross Motor Function Classification System (GMFCS); data from the Ontario Motor Growth Study (Rosenbaum et al. 2002). Kendall's tau-b (limb involvement in four categories: hemiplegia, diplegia, triplegia and quadriplegia by GMFCS)=0.13, p=0.001. Pearson's χ^2 test (limb involvement in four categories: hemiplegia, diplegia, triplegia and quadriplegia by GMFCS), p<0.001. Published with permission from Gorter et al. (2004).

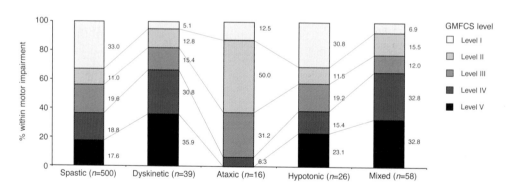

Figure 4.4 Distribution of 'type of motor impairment' by Gross Motor Function Classification System (GMFCS); data from the Ontario Motor Growth study (Rosenbaum et al. 2002). Pearson's χ^2 test (motor impairment by GMFCS), p<0.001. Published with permission from Gorter et al. (2004).

by therapists who have been trained to use the GMFM in a standardized way. It is widely applied in both clinical evaluations and research, and is available in several languages.

However, what the GMFM was never intended to do was to evaluate the *quality* of motor control of young people with CP. An initial approach to address that goal was the development of the Gross Motor Performance Measure (GMPM) (Boyce et al. 1991,1995).

Although the GMPM has been used occasionally (Thomas et al. 2001; Buckon et al. 2004), it is complicated to administer and covers only a subset of the GMFM items for which qualitative assessment is needed.

Work is now under way to redesign, simplify and complete the GMPM under the new and more appropriate title of 'Quality FM' (Wright, 2011, personal communication). This name reflects the idea that the new measure is an effort to capture aspects of the quality of performance of the GMFM items that look at standing, walking, running and jumping. Using the analogy of a microscope with several lenses of varying strength, it is expected that the Quality FM will provide a useful 'high-power' view of the qualitative aspects of function of people with CP once they have achieved the ability to do the activities in these dimensions of the GMFM. This in turn will enable service providers to target and measure interventions directed at specific aspects of function and quality of function in young people with CP.

References

Bax M, Tydeman C, Flodmark O (2006) Clinical and MRI correlates of cerebral palsy: the European Cerebral Palsy Study. *JAMA* 296: 1602–8.

Bleck EE (1987) *Orthopaedic Management in Cerebral Palsy. Clinics in Developmental Medicine No. 99/100.* Oxford: Blackwell Scientific Publications Ltd.

Boyce W, Gowland C, Hardy S et al. (1991) Development of a Quality of Movement Measure for children with cerebral palsy. *Phys Ther* 71: 820–32.

Boyce W, Gowland C, Rosenbaum P et al. (1995) The Gross Motor Performance Measure: validity and responsiveness of a measure of quality of movement. *Phys Ther* 75: 603–13.

Buckon CE, Thomas SS, Piatt JH Jr, Aiona MD, Sussman MD (2004) Selective dorsal rhizotomy versus orthopedic surgery: a multidimensional assessment of outcome efficacy. *Arch Phys Med Rehabil* 85: 457–65.

Cans C (2000) Surveillance of cerebral palsy in Europe: a collaboration of cerebral palsy surveys and registers. *Dev Med Child Neurol* 42: 816–24.

Colver A, Sethumadhavan T (2003) The term diplegia should be abandoned. *Arch Dis Child* 88: 286–90.

Eliasson AC, Krumlinde Sundholm L, Rösblad B et al (2006) The Manual Ability Classification System (MACS) for children with cerebral palsy: scale development and evidence of validity and reliability. *Dev Med Child Neurol* 48: 549–54.

Gorter JW, Rosenbaum PL, Hanna SE et al. (2004) Limb distribution, type of motor disorder and functional classification of cerebral palsy: how do they relate? *Dev Med Child Neurol* 46: 461–7.

Heinen F, Schröder AS, Döderlein L et al. (2009) Grafikgestützter Konsensus für die Behandlung von Bewegungsstörungen bei Kindern mit bilateralen spastischen Zerebralparesen (BS-CP). Graphically based Consensus on the treatment of movement disorders in children with bilateral spastic cerebral palsy (BS-CP). Therapiekurven – CP-Motorik Motor treatment curves in CP. *Monatsschr Kinderheilkd* 157: 789–94.

Hidecker MJC, Paneth N, Rosenbaum PL et al. (2011) Developing and validating the Communication Function Classification System (CFCS) for individuals with cerebral palsy. *Dev Med Child Neurol* 53: 704–10.

McCormick A, Brien M, Plourde J, Wood E, Rosenbaum P, McLean J (2007) The stability of the Gross Motor Function Classification System in adults with cerebral palsy. *Dev Med Child Neurol* 49: 265–9.

Morris C (2008) Development of the GMFCS (1997). *Dev Med Child Neurol* 50: 5.

Morris C, Kurinczuk JJ, Fitzpatrick R, Rosenbaum PL (2006) Reliability of the Manual Ability Classification System in the UK. *Dev Med Child Neurol* 48: 950–3.

Palisano R, Rosenbaum P, Walter S, Russell D, Wood E, Galuppi B (1997) Development and reliability of a system to classify gross motor function in children with cerebral palsy. *Dev Med Child Neurol* 39: 214–23.

Palisano R, Cameron D, Rosenbaum PL, Walter SD, Russell D (2006) Stability of the Gross Motor Function Classification System. *Dev Med Child Neurol* 48: 424–8.

Palisano RJ, Rosenbaum P, Bartlett D, Livingston MH (2008) Content validity of the expanded and revised Gross Motor Function Classification System. *Dev Med Child Neurol* 50: 744.

Rosenbaum PL, Walter SD, Hanna SE et al. (2002) Prognosis for gross motor function in cerebral palsy: creation of motor development curves. *JAMA* 288: 1357–63.

Rosenbaum PL, Palisano RJ, Bartlett DJ, Galuppi BE, Russell DJ (2008) Developing the Gross Motor Function Classification System for cerebral palsy: lessons and implications for classifying function in childhood disability. *Dev Med Child Neurol* 50: 249–53.

Russell, D, Rosenbaum PL, Avery L, Lane M (2002) *The Gross Motor Function Measure. GMFM-66 and GMFM-88 (Users' Manual). Clinics in Developmental Medicine No. 159.* London: Mac Keith Press.

Russman BS, Ashwal S (2004) Evaluation of the child with cerebral palsy. *Semin Pediatr Neurol* 11: 47–57.

Sanger TD, Delgado MR, Gaebler-Spira D, Hallett M, Mink JW (2003) Task Force on Childhood Motor Disorders. Classification and definition of disorders causing hypertonia in childhood. *Pediatrics* 111: e89–97.

Sanger TD, Chen D, Fehlings DL et al. (2010) Definition and classification of hyperkinetic movements in childhood. *Mov Disord* 25: 1538–49.

Steenbergen B, Meulenbroek RG (2006) Deviations in upper-limb function of the less-affected side in congenital hemiparesis. *Neuropsychologia* 44: 2296–307.

Thomas SS, Buckon CE, Phillips DS, Aiona MD, Sussman MD (2001) Interobserver reliability of the gross motor performance measure: preliminary results. *Dev Med Child Neurol* 43: 97–102.

Wood E, Rosenbaum P (2000) The Gross Motor Function Classification System for cerebral palsy: a study of reliability and stability over time. *Dev Med Child Neurol* 42: 292–6.

Chapter 5

What does the designation 'cerebral palsy' tell us, and how does this relate to other developmental and neurological disabilities?

Overview

In this chapter we discuss the many ways that people with cerebral palsy (CP) may be affected by underlying brain impairments and the 'secondary' consequences of developmental challenges. We draw parallels between CP and autism spectrum disorders to remind people that both conditions are really groups of phenomenologically defined developmental disabilities. We ponder the question of whether the term 'CP' has outlived its usefulness, and discuss why we believe that there is utility in retaining this term.

It will have become apparent in Chapter 1 that the term 'CP' describes a group of persisting, non-progressive conditions in the development of motor control that appear very early in life. Whatever impression the term 'CP' might convey, it is a label of convenience and not a single condition, let alone a specific 'disease'. What everyone with CP has in common are difficulties in the development of motor function that date from very early in life, resulting from impairments in the development and function of the immature central nervous system (CNS).

It seems likely that only a small minority of people with CP have a motor disorder as their sole impairment. Quantification of the extent of this minority is difficult. This is in part because of the reality that the extent of impairment of, for example, social or cognitive functioning and many other developmental challenges that may be seen in this population have not been explored systematically and are therefore not accurately known. It is likely that people with less complex levels of disability may not be identified as belonging to the 'population' of people with CP. This is because clinicians usually have a skewed experience of most conditions, in so far as people with more 'severe' difficulties are more likely to come to professional attention. Thus, there is often a tendency to assume that children with CP have other problems, to look for and identify these using norm-referenced measures and then to catalogue any variations of 'normal' function as 'problems' whether or not these observed differences are functionally important to the people identified as having them.

Nevertheless, it is usually the case that whatever factors are associated with the genesis of the CP will have affected other areas of the CNS. It is thus not surprising that people with CP can be expected to experience other 'neurodevelopmental' challenges of varying degree, particularly those listed in the second sentence of the 2007 definition of CP (Rosenbaum et al. 2007; see Chapter 1). We believe that it is therefore extremely important to be wary of judging the book by the cover. From a clinical perspective it is essential that each person's specific amalgam of skills and challenges be assessed and managed individually, rather than be based on some assumptions about what 'these people' are able/unable to do.

We would also emphasize that it is far too easy to assume that every disability or health challenge faced by people with CP is either a consequence of the impairment of brain development (the impairment that 'caused' the CP) or a secondary effect of these impairments (issues such as orthopaedic problems, nutritional compromise and growth limitations). We want to remind readers that, like the rest of the population, people with CP can develop health problems not related to their CP. (We are reminded of a young woman we met with Gross Motor Function Classification System [GMFCS] level IV CP whose acute gall bladder disease took weeks to be correctly recognized and managed appropriately because the treating physicians assumed her abdominal pain was part of her CP.) It is therefore very important to assess each health situation individually and not to make any assumptions about its aetiology until thoughtful evaluation of the problem has been completed.

On the other hand, for epidemiological purposes it can be very useful to describe the array of abilities and needs of a regional or national population. For example, knowing that children and young people in different GMFCS levels have importantly varying risks of hip migration and dislocation (Soo et al. 2006; Hägglund et al. 2007) or visual problems (Ghasia et al. 2008) can help practitioners, service managers and policy planners to estimate at a regional (population) level the need for orthopaedic/radiological or ophthalmological services, respectively. The work of colleagues in Northern Ireland has illustrated how one can identify broad levels of the functional needs of a population of children and young people with CP (Parkes et al. 2005).

Kennes et al. (2002) and Saigal et al. (2005) have reported the prevalence of a number of functional issues by 'severity' of motor difficulties categorized by the Gross Motor

Function Classification System (GMFCS) (Palisano et al. 1997, 2008). These reports illustrate the varying rates of functional impairments in different spheres of development and show that there is no automatic correspondence between one aspect of functional limitation (e.g. in motor activity) and other aspects of child development. In addition, while there is a correlation between some aspects of health-related quality of life (meaning functional status) and the level of motor difficulty, there are no systematic variations in self-reported 'quality of life' by GMFCS level (Rosenbaum et al. 2007). These findings (discussed in more detail in Chapter 12) illustrate how important it is to be clear and specific about whether, and how, the 'severity' of CP is a determinant of other aspects of functional well-being.

Against this background, it has often been argued, particularly by medical clinicians working in this field, that the term 'CP', or even the use of phrases such as 'the cerebral palsies' or the 'CP syndromes', should be abandoned or downgraded. A paper to this effect has been published by Bax et al. (2007). In that report, the authors suggested that using the term 'CP' may lead to a failure to explore and detail the full range of impairments seen in affected individuals, that the pathogenesis of the underlying problems will not be considered or sought and that interventions may not always be appropriate. We agree with the concern, but do not agree that abandoning the label 'CP' is an answer to these important issues. This is discussed more fully below.

It is also suggested that historical names and eponyms in other circumstances are now no more than curiosities. Examples such as Saint Vitus dance, mongolism, idiot, imbecile and moron readily come to mind, and it is argued that it follows that it would be equally appropriate now to abandon the term 'CP'. This approach is understandable, and if one were starting from scratch to describe and explore 'CP' as a newly described entity, then this idea could possibly be implemented.

There are, however, major obstacles to such an approach. The first is that, unlike many specific conditions, CP does not have a unified discrete cause or pathology in terms of it being a genetic disorder or an inborn error of metabolism. Nor is there a clear and consistent pathway by which it develops. It follows that there is no individual named disorder that can replace the term. Being aware of the distinctions between a specific 'disease' and a neurodevelopmental condition will serve both parents and professionals well.

Next is the reality that not only does the term CP have an historical context, but also its use has continued to date. A major implication of this fact is that there are a large number of impressive epidemiological studies that have been important in their own right. They have helped to characterize the condition, including identifying possible causal pathways (e.g. associations of CP with prematurity, rhesus incompatibility, twinning, maternal infection, maternal iodine deficiency). These studies have also been essential for service planning and delivery. Many of these studies are continuing and include rigorous criteria that determine what data are collected and counted.

Should the notion of 'CP' be abandoned, the potential loss of information from these studies would have an adverse effect on future health care and other provisions for people with CP. It is also relevant that use of the term 'CP' extends beyond the professional community. We have in mind bodies such as the United Cerebral Palsy Association in the USA and Scope in the UK. These and other organizations focus on CP in terms of service provision, advocacy and research across the lifespan.

It is also appropriate to argue that it is now exceptional for either lay people or professionals to hold the simplistic view that CP is a single entity. As has been detailed in Chapter 1, both past and current definitions emphasize the diversity of the clinical spectra that are seen.

In illustrating this point it is useful to draw an analogy between CP and the host of related conditions that are aggregated under the label of autistic spectrum disorder (ASD) or 'pervasive developmental disorder'. The commonly used term ASD clearly implies that there is a potential range ('spectrum') of clinical features of varying severity and indeed with differing emphases with respect to clinical features. It is also accepted that ASDs can be seen in association with a wide variety of structural brain impairments but that, to a greater frequency than is seen in CP, structural brain impairments may not be demonstrable. Despite a number of genetic studies, it is recognized that at present there is no unifying pathogenetic mechanism for ASDs.

Like CP, autism is an evolving and life-long disorder. Again, as in CP, changes in presentation and severity of impact can occur with age. This is illustrated, for example, by the development in some young people of epilepsy and the emergence of other mental health symptomatology over the developing years of childhood and adolescence. Based on this analogy it is appropriate to argue for the retention of the term CP in the same way as it is appropriate to argue for the retention of the term ASD as two examples of prevalent and challenging developmental disabilities.

The many and varied ASDs are often talked about as if they were a unitary 'disease', when in fact they can manifest in protean ways and have enormously varied impacts on the lives of the young people who have them and on their caregivers. It is also instructive to learn that in the proposed fifth edition of the Diagnostic and Statistical Manual of the American Psychiatric Association, the many labels associated with subtypes of autism will almost certainly be abandoned in favour of a single 'condition' with subgroups, as is the case now with CP.

It is also helpful to examine other groups of neurological disorders, for example the epilepsies, learning disabilities (DSM-IV usage: mental retardation), communication disorders and sensory impairments, in order to make the point that CP is over-represented in these populations when contrasted with a population of typically developing children. Here the links occur not only because of there being common or overlapping neuropathologies, but also because both CP and other neurological disorders have the potential to produce effects beyond the hallmark features that distinguish that condition (motor impairment in CP and social communication disorders in ASDs). These are often referred to as 'secondary' manifestations of the disorder. It is important to be aware that, in addition to the 'brain impairments' that underlie all of these neuro-developmental disabilities, there is an increased likelihood that children will experience restricted opportunities for social involvement, potentially leading to secondary limitations in 'participation' (engagement in life).

A further parallel can be drawn with traumatic and other acquired brain injury in children. Here affected individuals can ultimately present with the same range of impairments as are seen in CP. In the case of children with traumatic brain injury, the clinical presentations and challenges can be very different depending on the age, extent and severity of injury, premorbid personality and many other factors.

As has been indicated in Chapter 1, one of the loose ends with the definition of CP is the upper age limit that is appropriate to apply when describing a disorder that affects the immature brain as being 'CP'. Although we are aware that it is arbitrary, it is our view that it would not be appropriate to include the effects of traumatic brain injury in children as an example of CP when the injury has occurred after the first 2 years of life. In part this is an approach determined by convention. In the larger part, however, the significance of a period of normal neurological development on later functioning (when children sustain acquired brain injuries after the early years of life) makes for sufficient differences in clinical presentation, effects on the individual and family, interventions and outcomes for it to be unhelpful in the majority of cases to regard such individuals' disabilities as examples of 'CP'.

At the same time, of course, the impact of a brain injury acquired early in life on a child's development and on the child's family is really quite similar, regardless of the specific timing of the traumatic injury. It is this reality that makes many of these age-related distinctions difficult and at times somewhat arbitrary.

There are enough common features between CP and traumatic brain injury for there to be very similar principles in terms of how individuals are likely to progress, on the clinical approaches that are required for assessment and for helpful intervention, on the effects on families and on the long-term outlook. So far as clinical service provision is concerned, it would be reasonable to anticipate that this should complement the approach to services provided to children with CP and their families. Conversely, it would not be appropriate to regard these two patterns of neurological disability as competing with one another for relevant resources.

The distinctions between 'CP' and an acquired brain injury that produces phenotypically similar findings are important for epidemiological considerations. Also, self-evidently, the mechanisms of acquired brain injury, and efforts at prevention, are importantly different from these same efforts in 'CP'.

Based on this review of practice, it follows that the authors of this book are firmly of the view that it is appropriate to continue to use the term CP but to use it in the full realization of its limitations as well as its advantages.

References

Bax MCO, Flodmark O, Tydeman C (2007) Definition and classification of cerebral palsy. From syndrome toward disease. *Dev Med Child Neurol* 49 (Suppl. 109): 39–41.

Ghasia F, Brunstrom J, Gordon M, Tychsen L (2008) Frequency and severity of visual sensory and motor deficits in children with cerebral palsy: gross motor function classification scale. *Invest Ophthalmol Vis Sci* 49: 572–80.

Hägglund G, Lauge-Pedersen H, Wagner P (2007) Characteristics of children with hip displacement in cerebral palsy. *BMC Musculoskelet Disord* 8: 101.

Kennes J, Rosenbaum P, Hanna S et al. (2002) Health status of school-aged children with cerebral palsy: information from a population-based sample. *Dev Med Child Neurol* 44: 240–7.

Palisano R, Rosenbaum P, Walter S, Russell D, Wood E, Galuppi B (1997) Development and reliability of a system to classify gross motor function in children with cerebral palsy. *Dev Med Child Neurol* 39: 214–23.

Palisano RJ, Rosenbaum P, Bartlett D, Livingston MH (2008) Content validity of the expanded and revised Gross Motor Function Classification System. *Dev Med Child Neurol* 50: 744.

Parkes J, Dolk H, Hill N (2005) *Cerebral Palsy in Children and Young Adults in Northern Ireland (Birth years 1977–1997): A Comprehensive Report.* Belfast: Queen's University Belfast.

Rosenbaum PL, Livingston MH, Palisano RJ, Galuppi BE, Russell DJ (2007) Quality of life and health-related quality of life of adolescents with cerebral palsy. *Dev Med Child Neurol* 49: 516–21.

Saigal S, Rosenbaum P, Stoskopf B et al. (2005) Development, reliability and validity of a new measure of overall health for pre-school children. *Qual Life Res* 14: 241–55.

Soo B, Howard JJ, Boyd RN et al. (2006) Hip displacement in cerebral palsy. *J Bone Joint Surg Am* 88: 121–9.

Part 2

Contextual factors and critical thinking

Chapter 6

Evaluating evidence

Overview

The parents of children with cerebral palsy (CP) ask a host of common and fundamental questions about their child's situation, the answers to which are very important to them. This chapter provides a brief primer on ways of thinking about the evidence – an approach that is often called 'critical appraisal'. This set of ideas is designed simply to alert readers to the importance of bringing a thoughtful and analytically critical approach to all our appraisals of the literature about any aspect of CP. We want to indicate that as consumers (whether we are parents or service providers looking at the 'evidence') we should be cautious about the claims people make about the natural history of people with CP, about treatment, about what we measure as outcomes or about causation. We also argue that as researchers we need to design and execute studies with appropriate attention to the methodological details so that the findings of our work can stand up to the critical scrutiny of colleagues and families.

Few people would question how to manage acute appendicitis in an ill child: the surgeon is called in and the offending appendix is removed. Alas, in any field where there is no clear and proven way to do things (as is true for most decisions in CP), there is usually an 'inverse' rule, where the number of approaches varies according to the degree of uncertainty about the value and 'truth' of any specific one.

It is important to identify openly the tensions that exist between researchers and people who want answers immediately. It takes time to acquire solid evidence that the things we do actually 'work', and people who want help immediately can appear as impatient. It is wholly understandable that people with CP, their families, caring professionals and indeed society at large want to effect improvements, if not a cure, by whatever means seem to make sense to them, and as quickly as possible. There will always be varied approaches to the management of conditions where there is no proven cure, and usually a degree of controversy arises whenever unproven therapies are debated. This is certainly the case in the treatment and management of CP, where old traditions are constantly being challenged by people promoting new ways to think and act. One of the big challenges for both service providers and parents is to evaluate claims about therapies, both old and new.

Many of the issues addressed in this book – for example what causes CP and what interventions may be helpful – are based on available evidence from a combination of experience and research. We recognize that parents, service providers and people who make health and social service policies all want to act in the most responsible manner, using 'evidence' on which to base their decisions. In this chapter we feel it is useful to examine how evidence can be evaluated in the context of there being what many would regard as a limited number of 'proven' scientific data. Specifically, how can we evaluate and make decisions about new ideas and unproven claims about issues of causation or treatment of CP?

As either service providers or parents we are expected to know how to make sense of the claims that are often made by people who have a particular approach to 'treatment'. That approach may be based on a specific view of what CP is, or how it happens, or how the brain functions and 'recovers', and so on. The information about treatment effectiveness is available in a myriad of media. We hear things on the radio and television or from friends and family, we read articles in newspapers and magazines, and of course the Internet is an inexhaustible source of 'information'. We may often be unsure whether what is being reported applies to our child or our patient, whether the treatment is available in our community or from our service, and how much it might cost in money, time and effort. (For examples of how people evaluate these issues, both generally and specifically, see Rosenbaum [1995], Rosenbaum et al. [2001] and Rosenbaum and Stewart [2003a,b].) Specific issues requiring consideration under this heading are discussed more fully in Chapter 10.

How then does one make sense of what might at times be conflicting information and 'evidence', or might simply sound too good to be true? Educators who teach research methods have written excellent articles and texts (e.g. Sackett et al. 1991) to help people become informed consumers of the emerging claims and 'evidence'. These resources provide a critical lens through which to view the constantly changing picture of claims and research findings.

Before we discuss the many ways that people offer therapy for children with CP, we have tried, in this section of the book, to provide an overview of how readers can be thoughtful and critical in evaluating any claims about treatment. We have done this by addressing a few of the most common questions that both parents and front-line service providers ask – or should ask – about the things they hear. These are also the questions we ourselves ask when new ideas are being promoted. We subscribe to the view that if it sounds too good to be true, then it probably is. And we remind ourselves that a single case report does not constitute proof of the generalizability and effectiveness of that intervention for other people in other circumstances (for, as a wise person once said, 'The plural of anecdote is not "evidence".').

One other cautionary comment is important: the 'absence of evidence' is not the same as 'evidence of absence' (of the effectiveness of treatment). In a relatively young academic field like the scientific study of CP, much work remains to be done to discover the best approaches to treatment and management. Much of what we 'know' is based on less than perfect evidence, so we often must make decisions for our patients (or our own children) with the best of what is available. Nonetheless, by becoming critical thinkers and asking thoughtful questions, we believe that everyone involved in the care and management, and the raising, of children with CP will do a better job.

Where have we come from?

Biomedicine in the twentieth century was grounded in a tradition of scientific enquiry that led to what has now become widely known as 'evidence-based medicine' (EBM). In contrast to 'eminence-based medicine' (the old tradition of professorial pontification), EBM is built on a base of scientific research that, at its best, has been undertaken using sound methodological principles that are thought to lead to credible findings (Sackett et al. 1991). Among the most scientifically well-grounded foundations of clinical medicine are areas such as cardiology and oncology, where large randomized trials and multiyear prospective longitudinal studies have provided evidence about issues such as the natural history of conditions, determinants of outcome and of course the benefits (or not) of specific interventions.

The academic field of childhood disability is, by contrast, much younger in its development. As a result, the evidence base for the things we believe and 'know' is less well established. Much of our current knowledge is empirical, built on the experience of thoughtful practitioners, although more recently there is an emerging body of credible scientific study becoming available to guide practice. Needless to say, the whole field is constantly evolving, and the evidence presented in this book will, sooner or later, become outdated and give way to newer and presumably stronger research findings.

For this reason, this section of the text is designed to help readers become critical 'consumers' of the literature. Our intention is to whet people's appetite for how best to separate the wheat from the chaff and to identify both the potential strengths and limitations of any research that addresses the issues of major interest to people concerned with childhood disability. For ease of access, several major themes are presented, each related to a question that might be asked as one begins to evaluate the research that addresses the things we do. While not a primer on research methods, these concepts will hopefully prove useful to many readers.

The clinical question asks: *What do we know about the 'natural history' of development of children with CP? What can we expect to see over time?*

The critical appraisal issues ask: *How sound was the research design that led to the 'evidence' that people are using?* and *How representative is the sample being reported?*

The best way to answer a question about the natural history of any condition is to assemble a 'representative' group of people with that condition (technically called a 'cohort') whose progress is followed systematically over 'real' (calendar) time. The primary outcomes of interest should have been identified before the study began, and the outcomes should then have been measured appropriately with the 'right' instruments.

In fact, it is usually extremely difficult to find a 'virgin' population of people with the condition of interest who have not had any intervention. Even if such a cohort could be assembled, it would not represent today's reality in many parts of the world. In almost all cases, people with the conditions of interest are identified and 'treated' by whatever combination of services is currently available. One is therefore more likely to be talking about the 'unnatural history' of most conditions of interest.

What do we mean by a 'representative' sample? This idea refers to a group of people who are selected on the basis of having the condition of interest, which ought to have been carefully defined before the study begins. For example, in a study of the 'natural history' of CP, it is essential that the researchers undertaking the study have specified what exactly they mean by 'CP', including the age at which children are 'confirmed' to have it, and have defined their inclusion and exclusion criteria (see Rosenbaum et al. [2002] as an example of such a study). The cohort should include the full spectrum of 'cases' rather than just those who were specially selected because they have some particular characteristic that makes them easily identifiable or 'interesting'. In other words, the cohort must not be made up simply of people who have the most or least severe forms of disability, or particular features such as the presence or absence of additional developmental disorders such as epilepsy or learning disabilities (DSM-IV usage: mental retardation).

The requirement for a representative sample concerns our expectation that we will be able to be confident that the findings of the study are relevant and applicable to the questions we have about the population of people with CP with whom we work. In other words, we need to know that the research findings on which we rely involved people similar to those to whom we will apply the research findings. If we work with people with the full range of abilities and limitations, we need to know that the information on which we are basing our predictions was assembled and assessed in the same way as we do things.

One difficulty with cohort studies is that they are often assembled from among the people seen in the clinic where the researchers work. Why might this be an issue? The reason is that the people with the condition whom we see more frequently are often importantly different from those with the condition whom we see less often or not at all. Depending on where and how the cohort is assembled, the nature of that group might therefore vary considerably from what is 'representative' of the whole universe of people with that condition.

Imagine, for example, whom one might see in a CP orthopaedic clinic. Unless that service systematically follows *every* child with CP in the community, it is very likely that there will be a significant skew towards children with more 'severe' involvement of their CP, at least as categorized by GMFCS level (e.g. Parkes et al. 2006). These are, after all, the people who orthopaedic surgeons would be asked to see. It has been reported (Soo et al. 2006; Hägglund et al. 2007) that the proportion of children and young people with CP who have problems with hip 'migration' increases virtually linearly across GMFCS levels. Thus, the children and young people in a CP orthopaedic clinic are necessarily (and appropriately) skewed towards the more functionally compromised end of the clinical spectrum. Therefore, in reporting hip problems in children with CP we would get different rates from orthopaedic clinics and population surveys that included 'everyone' with CP.

A similar issue would be a concern regarding the 'outcomes' of young people with CP. Until recently, few programmes have provided systematic assessment and follow-up of adolescents with CP, so we are likely to know about, selectively recall and be able to find those who present to a clinic with problems – of pain, loss of function, contractures, mental health worries, etc. We may too easily forget about the people who are not coming to clinic – perhaps because their lives are progressing well, perhaps because they have no confidence in our ability to be helpful . . . Whatever the reasons they are 'lost to follow-up', we miss the opportunity to include their life perspectives in the information we collect and report, and thus easily end up with a biased (systematically skewed) sample from which we may draw inappropriate conclusions about the whole population.

The best information about (un)natural history will come from well-designed studies that have assembled their cohorts using population-based samples and then followed them forward over time to evaluate the outcomes of interest. Such cohorts will often be found through population-based registries of people with the condition. The Surveillance of Cerebral Palsy in Europe (SCPE) (Cans 2000) represents such a collection of data. (The SCPE is described in a bit more detail in Chapter 4.) The assumption is that all the children within the catchment area of the case register have been identified systematically, and, whether they are receiving services or not, are potentially equally available to be included in studies of the outcomes of interest (see, for example, Dickinson et al. [2007] and Fauconnier et al. [2009]). In fact, with registers that are thought to be comprehensive, it is possible to assess the extent to which the samples one actually recruits are, or are not, representative of the larger population from which the sample is drawn (Morris et al. 2004, 2006).

The clinical question asks: *How can we assess whether a treatment or intervention does more good than harm?*

The critical appraisal issues ask: *How is treatment effectiveness established?* and *What outcomes were measured?*

Children with CP usually receive a host of intervention services over many years. These are provided on the basis of our beliefs about the effectiveness of each modality of treatment, bolstered to a greater or lesser degree by evidence from the literature. Such evidence might have been drawn from case reports and case series. It hopefully will also include methodologically sound clinical trial research that has been designed to account for potential biases in the way the studies were conducted. What are the differences between these types of studies, and why do they matter? These questions address several essential underpinnings of clinical intervention research and are considered briefly here.

It is important to recognize at the outset of any discussion about the effects of treatment that in essence we are always trying to discern 'cause and effect' connections (Rosenbaum and Law 1996). We provide an intervention (the cause), we look at the 'outcome' (the effect) and we make an assumption that the changes we observe were 'caused by' the treatment. On the surface this seems to be a clear and logical thought process. Why then are things not always so simple? What are the possible 'threats to validity' of these observations that cause us to pause and reflect?

There are several considerations in answering this question. The first is that, in any situation where time is an element of the story (as is the case when the effects of treatments are being assessed over weeks or months, and often years), there may be other processes at work 'in the background' that influence the outcomes. In children, the most obvious process is natural development, something that must be recognized to happen to children with CP as it does to all other children. The interventions we provide are offered to people (children) whose natural tendency is to grow and change as time passes. Our research challenge, therefore, is to separate the 'active ingredients' of our treatments from the influences of natural development in order to detect the 'signal' (of treatment-induced change) from the background 'noise' of other possible influences on that change.

A related idea is that whatever treatment we are interested to assess is almost certainly being provided as just one of several intervention activities. If we focus too closely on the 'foreground' (looking only at that treatment), we may easily forget to consider what else is going on in the 'background' (i.e. the other activities and treatments that are also happening). In that circumstance, we may draw the conclusion that it was our treatment that made the observable difference, when in fact it was another factor, or perhaps a combination of factors working together, that was responsible for the changes. Readers interested in exploring this issue more closely may want to look at a case report by Joyce and Clark (1996) and the accompanying commentary by Rosenbaum and Law (1996).

It is also helpful to remember that just because one event follows another does not mean that the former *caused* the latter. As noted briefly in Chapter 1, in law this concept is known as 'post hoc ergo propter hoc' ('after that, therefore because of that'). There is a witticism that 'All heroin addicts started on milk', but no-one would attribute drug addiction to milk exposure. It is therefore important to understand that separating out the effects of the things we do in treatment from the other influences in a child's life is more challenging than is sometimes recognized.

How can these 'threats to validity' be overcome? The strongest evidence about the effects of treatments comes from 'human experiments'. The randomized control trial (RCT) is usually cited as the pinnacle of evidence for the effects of any intervention. When these studies are carried out with sound randomization methodology, and include appropriately large samples of randomly selected 'cases', when they measure the right things and when they control as many as possible of the potential biases described above, one can have more confidence that the findings are likely to be valid. Why then is there such a dearth of RCT-based evidence in the field of childhood disability?

The cleanest RCTs ask a focused question about a specific aspect of human health, evaluate the effectiveness of a particular targeted intervention, have a credible comparison 'treatment' and assess a discrete outcome. Drug trials of medications to lower blood pressure are an example of such a relatively 'clean' study. People with defined levels of elevated blood pressure are randomly assigned to receive a new treatment or a comparison intervention (usually a conventional management strategy). The primary outcome (a prespecified degree of blood pressure control) is measured after a predefined period of time and side effects are assessed; a conclusion can then be drawn about how the new treatment compares with the contrast intervention and whether the benefits outweigh the risks.

With interventions for children with developmental disabilities like CP, it is often very difficult to bring the same degree of control to the RCT 'experiment'. The interventions are often not as specific and discrete as a drug treatment (although studies with botulinum toxin are a notable exception). The time course of the interventions and their effects is usually months or years rather than weeks (as might be the case in a hypertension study, at least for the immediate effects). Other treatments and activities are going on in the lives of children with CP and their families that can make the provision of the new treatment challenging and the interpretation of outcomes difficult. Despite the prevalence of CP, there is often a major difficulty in finding large enough numbers of children who fit the inclusion and exclusion criteria for the study. In selecting who is suitable for inclusion in any specific study, one almost always excludes some people, and this necessary research step then has implications for the eventual generalizability of the findings. Finally, assessing the outcomes of interventions may pose challenges, both because the right tools may not be available (discussed below) and because the outcomes of interest are not as clear and specific as a predefined lowering of blood pressure. These issues have been addressed briefly by Rosenbaum (2010).

An alternative approach to the human experiment, one that lends itself well to interventions in children with CP, is the multiple-baseline single-participant study. The excellent studies of Butler (1986), Bower and McLellan (1994) and Bower et al. (1996) provide clear illustrations of how this can be done. With this design we assess the functions of interest on several occasions to establish the pattern of change that is happening 'natu-rally' before the intervention. We then begin the intervention, and rather than making single before–after observations, we measure the same functional outcomes on several occasions during and following treatment. Preferably, people who are 'blind' to the details of the intervention should do this. We are looking for an unbiased assessment of change in the patterns of development of that function after the onset of treatment. If this approach to the evaluation of an intervention is repeated with several individu-als, if clear goals are specified and if the timing of the onset of treatment is randomly assigned, one may then be able to discern consistent patterns of effects across individual children using that intervention and draw conclusions that are more credible than single case reports.

The main message regarding the evaluation of claims about the effectiveness of any treatment is that the more carefully a study is designed and executed, the more confi-dence one can have in the credibility of the findings from that research. On the other hand, the more the findings of a study can be challenged with respect to possible biases in the design of the research, who is included and excluded, how the outcomes were assessed and reported, and the analyses that are done, the less comfortable one will be with the believability of the results or the applicability of the findings of that study to our own patients. This is why an anecdote or dramatic case report can at best provide grist for the research mill and further studies, but on their own ought never to be con-sidered credible evidence of the effectiveness of any treatment.

The clinical question asks: *How do we measure the 'right' things, and what are the best instruments?*

The critical appraisal issue asks: *How do we assess whether the measures we use are the right 'tools' for the assessment of outcomes?*

As described elsewhere (see Chapters 4 and 13), the measurement of outcomes depends on instruments that measure what we want to measure reliably (consistently) and pro-vide us with valid (true) and useful information. In evaluating the findings of research published in the literature, we need to know the answers to two specific questions.

First, were the outcomes that were measured the 'right' ones? For example, if an inter-vention is designed to improve mobility function, does the study clearly and validly report that outcome as a primary finding? At times people may unwittingly engage in what is known as the 'substitution game' and measure what they think matters, or what it is possible to measure, rather than what they originally planned to assess. They might do this because they believe that the things they choose to measure are the relevant pathophysiological underpinnings to the 'clinical' outcomes, and are therefore more important than the function results. Thus, for example, after a study of selective dorsal rhizotomy (a neurosurgical procedure that involves cutting nerves to decrease spastic-ity), performed to improve mobility, the investigators reported changes in the range of movement and improvement in spasticity scores (Peacock et al. 1987; Peacock and Staudt 1991). If the study does not provide information on changes in mobility, one is left uncertain about the impact of the intervention on the primary outcome of interest. Just because the 'impairments' have changed does not automatically mean that function has improved (Wright et al. 2008).

Second, to assess outcomes (particularly change over time in some aspect of function) one needs measures that have been validated to achieve that evaluative task. That means that the measures used have appropriately been shown to detect change when it happens and to demonstrate stability in the absence of meaningful change. Using the 'wrong' tools may lead one to conclude that a treatment was ineffective when in fact it may have been that the tools failed to detect the changes that happened (Rosenbaum et al. 1990).

Note, however, that there are many other reasons to measure things. One may want to have a systematic, descriptive account of people's function for which measures with the appropriate content will be used. These do not need to be change-detecting measures, but they have to be able to provide perspectives relevant to the question being asked. One may need to assess the extent to which a person 'measures up' against others, for which norm-referenced measures are needed. Examples would be assessments of height, weight or intelligence, where one is comparing the person being assessed against a population of people like that person. The basic considerations are: is the content of the measure what I wish to know, and is there evidence that the measure can do this 'job' (i.e. has it been demonstrated to be 'valid' to measure what I want to measure?)?

The clinical question asks: *What do we know about causation of CP?*

The critical appraisal issue asks: *How are causal connections established?*

In discussing the effectiveness of interventions, reference was made to the difficulty of establishing causality. This is a particularly challenging issue in medicine for a number of reasons. First, with respect to causation we recognize that there may be predisposing, precipitating, perpetuating and protective factors at work. Disentangling what these factors are, and their relative importance, can be very complex.

As but one example, we have traditionally believed that difficulties at the time of labour and delivery can lead to 'hypoxic–ischaemic encephalopathy' (brain damage from insufficient oxygen to the brain), which can in turn 'cause' CP (a classic example of 'post hoc ergo propter hoc'). However, modern imaging techniques have increasingly allowed experts to ascertain the nature and location of impairments to brain structure. In addition, new insights into neurobiology and particularly an understanding of the timing of central nervous system development have made it possible at times to 'date' the timing of the impairments of brain structure that are associated with CP.

With these advances it is now clear that some infants who experience perinatal difficulties *already* have impaired brain structure (and perhaps function as well). These impairments may have 'predisposed' these infants to difficulties in adaptation to the birthing process (the 'precipitating' factor) and immediate postnatal adjustments.

Because a brain impairment (a 'perpetuating' factor) may make it more difficult for an infant to cope with a biological 'insult', these infants may already have been more vulnerable to experiencing a deprivation of oxygen supply to the central nervous system, perhaps compounding the functional problems they experienced later. The child's eventual functional outcome could then reflect a combination of these forces, coupled with 'protective' factors such as rapid resuscitation in the perinatal period and family support, other developmental abilities that are inherent in this child's make-up, life opportunities, therapies and so on.

What can be seen with this scenario is that the notion of 'causation' is far more complex than was traditionally thought. In other words, the causal pathways are almost always more entangled and multidetermined than simple connections between an earlier 'event' and a later 'outcome'. Work in a number of centres around the world is making it possible to disentangle these 'causal pathways' (see Stanley et al. 2000) as a basis for preventative strategies that will, in future, hopefully allow more infants to avoid these complex biomedical challenges and develop smoothly.

References

Bower E, McLellan DL (1994) Evaluating therapy in cerebral palsy. *Child Care Health Dev* 20: 409–19.

Bower E, McLellan DL, Arney J, Campbell MJ (1996) A randomized controlled trial of different intensities of physiotherapy and different goal-setting procedures in 44 children with cerebral palsy. *Dev Med Child Neurol* 38: 226–37.

Butler C (1986) Effects of powered mobility on self-initiated behaviours of very young children with locomotor disability. *Dev Med Child Neurol* 28: 325–32.

Cans C. (2000) Surveillance of cerebral palsy in Europe: a collaboration of cerebral palsy surveys and registers. *Dev Med Child Neurol* 42: 816–24.

Dickinson HO, Parkinson KN, Ravens-Sipberer U et al. (2007) Self-reported quality of life of 8–12-year-old children with cerebral palsy: a cross-sectional European study. *Lancet* 369: 2171–8.

Fauconnier J, Dickinson HO, Beckung E et al. (2009) Participation in life situations of 8–12 year old children with cerebral palsy: cross sectional European study. *BMJ* 338: b1458.

Hägglund G, Lauge-Pedersen H, Wagner P (2007) Characteristics of children with hip displacement in cerebral palsy. *BMC Musculoskelet Disord* 8: 101.

Joyce P, Clark C (1996) The use of craniosacral therapy to treat gastroesophageal reflux in infants. *Infants Young Child* 9: 51–8.

Morris C, Galuppi BE, Rosenbaum PL (2004) Reliability of family report for the Gross Motor Function Classification System. *Dev Med Child Neurol* 46: 455–60.

Morris C, Kurinczuk JJ, Fitzpatrick R, Rosenbaum PL (2006) Who best to make the assessment? Professionals and families' classifications of gross motor function are highly consistent. *Arch Dis Child* 91: 675–9.

Parkes J, Kerr C, McDowell BC, Cosgrove AP (2006) Recruitment bias in a population-based study of children with cerebral palsy. *Pediatrics* 118: 1616–22.

Peacock WJ, Arens LJ, Berman B (1987) Cerebral palsy spasticity. Selective posterior rhizotomy. *Pediatr Neurosci* 13: 61–6.

Peacock WJ, Staudt LA (1991) Functional outcomes following selective posterior rhizotomy in children with cerebral palsy. *J Neurosurg* 74: 380–5.

Rosenbaum P (1995) Alternative treatments: thoughts from the trenches. Available at: http://www.canchild.ca/Default.aspx?tabid=110 (accessed 7 January 2008).

Rosenbaum P (2010) The randomized controlled trial: an excellent design, but can it address the big questions in neurodisability? *Dev Med Child Neurol* 52: 111.

Rosenbaum P, Law M (1996) Craniosacral therapy and gastroesophageal reflux: a commentary. *Infants Young Child* 9: 69–74.

Rosenbaum P, Stewart D (2003a) Alternative and complementary therapies for children and youth with brain injury – Part 1: controversies. Available at: http://www.canchild.ca/Default.aspx?tabid=111 (accessed 7 January 2008).

Rosenbaum P, Stewart D (2003b) Alternative and complementary therapies for children and youth with acquired brain injury – Part 2: finding and evaluating the evidence. Available at: http://www.canchild.ca/Default.aspx?tabid=536 (accessed 7 January 2008).

Rosenbaum PL, Cadman D, Russell D, Gowland C, Hardy S, Jarvis S (1990) Issues in measuring change in motor function in children with cerebral palsy. A special communication. *Phys Ther* 70: 125–31.

Rosenbaum P, Fehlings D, Iliffe C (2001) Hyperbaric oxygen therapy: hot or not? Available at: http://www.canchild.ca/Default.aspx?tabid=123 (accessed 7 January 2008).

Rosenbaum PL, Walter SD, Hanna SE et al. (2002) Prognosis for gross motor function in cerebral palsy: creation of motor development curves. *JAMA* 288: 1359–63.

Sackett DL, Haynes RB, Tugwell P. (1991) *Clinical Epidemiology: A Basic Science for Clinical Medicine*, 2nd edn. Boston: Little, Brown.

Soo B, Howard JJ, Boyd RN et al. (2006) Hip displacement in cerebral palsy. *J Bone Joint Surg Am* 88: 121–9.

Stanley FJ, Blair E, Alberman E (2000) *Cerebral Palsies: Epidemiology and Causal Pathways*. London: Mac Keith Press.

Wright FV, Rosenbaum PL, Goldsmith CH, Law M, Fehlings DL (2008) How do changes in body functions and structures, activity, and participation relate in children with cerebral palsy? *Dev Med Child Neurol* 50: 283–9.

Chapter 7

The International Classification of Functioning, Disability and Health

Overview

In 2001, the World Health Organization (WHO) published the International Classification of Functioning, Disability and Health. Known informally as the ICF, this framework for health has caught the attention of many people in the health field, perhaps most often those working in rehabilitation. This chapter presents the key concepts of the ICF, including the notions of capacity, performance and capability. It also highlights the ways that a person's environment influences what they do and how. We see this framework as a useful scaffold onto which we can 'rule in' relevant aspects of each child and family's strengths and needs. This in turn allows us to build a descriptive profile of each child and family's situation in order to identify 'points of entry' for action and to decide what aspects of the situation to measure as outcomes.

In 1980, WHO published the International Classification of Impairment, Disability and Handicap (ICIDH) (World Health Organization 1980). This original model of the consequences of a health issue was useful in reminding people that any 'condition' had biomedical components (at that time labelled 'impairments'), that these in turn could lead to functional limitations (called 'disabilities') and that the disabilities could impact on people's lives by restricting their life possibilities and cause 'handicaps'. Although the model illustrated a unidirectional left-to-right progression of these linked ideas, this way of thinking was, for many people, an important stimulus. It encouraged us to consider several components of the possible impact of a health condition on the person and to reflect on how to use these several dimensions in planning interventions (Rosenbaum 1998).

A revised and much improved framework resulted in the International Classification of Functioning, Disability and Health (World Health Organization 2001). The ICF emerged as a result of many years of international discussion and collaboration with, among others, disabled people (Fig. 7.1). The ICF incorporates modified versions of the original concepts: these include the structural and functional underpinnings of a condition (now collectively labelled 'body structure and function'), the impact of these impairments on 'activity' (what people can do and restrictions thereof) and the idea of 'participation' (engagement in life, and possible restrictions in this aspect of life). In addition, the contextual elements of 'personal factors' and 'environment' have been added to reflect the reality that, within a social model of disability, these factors, many of them outside the person, can be important determinants of whether or not a problem with body structure and function becomes a 'disabling' challenge (Rosenbaum 2007).

Note that the several components of this multivariable framework are all interconnected, illustrating that these concepts have a direct relationship with each other. In this respect the ICF can be considered a 'dynamic system', meaning that interventions or changes in one element of the system will very likely have impacts on other aspects of people's lives. Note as well that the language of the ICF is neutral rather than negative ('body structure and function' rather than 'impairment'; 'activity' instead of 'disability'; 'participation' instead of 'handicap').

To illustrate how the IFC can be used clinically for a case analysis for the individual person with cerebral palsy (CP), consider the case of Child 3.

Child 3
CC was a preterm-born infant, born at 28 weeks with a weight just under 1000g. She is now 6 years old and has bilateral spastic CP (Gross Motor Function Classification System [GMFCS] level IV; Manual Ability Classification System level II). She attends a

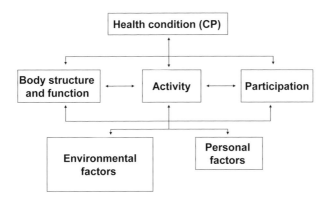

Figure 7.1 The World Health Organization International Classification of Functioning, Disability and Health framework.

disability class at a local school in a power wheelchair, where she is in an age-appropriate grade. Her general health is good, she hears and sees well with glasses, has never had seizures and is on no regular medication. She is partially dependent in activities of daily living (ADL), requiring help with dressing and accessing the toilet, but feeds herself and can access her computer on her own.

CC is the older of two children of a young couple. CC's mother usually attends clinic with her own mother (CC's maternal grandmother). CC is learning well in school and her teacher often has CC 'run down to the office' to deliver messages on behalf of the class. Outside school CC plays with her friends and is invited to birthday parties.

At a recent clinic visit, CC's mother took great delight in reporting the following anecdote: a few days earlier, CC's power wheelchair would not start. Her mother asked CC if, while playing with her friends in the garden, she had been riding the chair across the lawn and through the garden hose – which CC denied. Her mother then took the cover off the chair motor and water poured out. CC's mother grounded her daughter for a day for telling a lie – but told the story with great delight because she recognized both the 'mischief' her daughter had engaged in and the age-appropriate effort to cover up her 'crime'.

Consider CC's situation in ICF terms:

- At the level of *body structure and function*, CC has bilateral spastic CP, GMFCS level IV, associated with underlying periventricular leukomalacia. On examination she shows some evidence of contractures of her lower extremities, notable at hips, knees and ankles bilaterally but slightly more apparent on the left side. CC is in good health, has no apparent difficulties with sensory function and does not have seizures.

- At the level of *activity*, CC needs some help with ADLs but seeks opportunities to be as independent as she can. She has made progress in becoming capable with self-feeding and can undress her upper body, but needs help with trousers and underclothes. She is able to learn at an age-appropriate level.

- At the level of *participation* CC has friends and is given responsibilities at school by a teacher who had identified CC's capacity to accept the challenges associated with being the class messenger at times. The anecdote about the wheelchair breakdown illustrates CC's engagement with her friends in 'mischief' and the resultant social consequences associated with the adventure.

- At the level of *environmental factors*, CC lives in an intact family with a younger sister and considerable grandparental support. Her parents recognize and support the importance of fostering CC's capabilities, and have high expectations of her physical and social functioning in her family and immediate social circle. CC is able to attend her local school with a wheelchair-accessible regular class. CC's home has a garden in which she and her friends can play.

- At the level of *personal factors*, CC is clearly a socially popular and independent-minded child whose capability has been recognized by her class teacher. With parental encouragement – perhaps because they recognize her drive and her emerging abilities – CC is working at becoming as independent as possible.

This overview of CC's situation illustrates how a 'case analysis' can enable people – including parents as well as professionals – to identify elements of the person's situation. This makes it possible to create a profile of strengths and emerging abilities along with the problems in body structure and function that drew that individual to attention in the first place. In this (true-life) anecdote, the young family had come to appreciate their daughter's abilities and to encourage the emerging independence despite a significant degree of physical compromise that required her family and professionals to find other ways to foster her development.

Note that the notion of 'quality of life' is not part of the ICF framework. This is probably because the ICF is meant to provide an overview of the various components of a person's 'functioning' (the 'F' in ICF), whereas quality of life is an essentially personal valuation of one's status separate from the analytical profile described above. Quality of life issues are discussed in Chapter 12 on outcomes.

For parents and people working with youngsters with CP and other neurodisabilities, these concepts encourage us to think about interventions beyond the confines of 'treatment' of impairments in body structure and function implied by the original ICIDH framework (Rosenbaum and Stewart 2004). In many therapeutic traditions it was assumed (usually implicitly rather than formally) that one needed to remediate (and if possible 'fix') the basic problems of CP – for example, excess muscle tone, reflex abnormalities, obligatory motor patterns, etc. – if the person were to achieve 'normal' function. In fact, in some approaches children were actively discouraged from standing and walking 'abnormally', and as a consequence were perhaps restricted not only by their impairments but also by beliefs about how function would and should be achieved.

An alternative approach, and one to which we strongly subscribe, emphasizes the achievement of functional goals by whatever (safe) means possible. There is in fact some research evidence (Boyce et al. 1995) that children with CP need to learn basic 'functional' skills before they begin to improve the 'quality' of their movement patterns. This is of course developmentally consistent with the way that typically developing children learn to do things, such as cruise around furniture and 'toddle' before they become capable walkers later in the preschool years, and then are able to acquire the advanced 'skills' that allow them to ride a two-wheel bicycle or manoeuvre a skateboard.

Palisano (2006) has illustrated how the ICF allows us to identify all the relevant aspects of each person's situation as a basis for analysis of the factors that either constrain or perhaps enhance functional possibilities. This approach, which includes identifying a child's and family's strengths, is potentially far richer and more useful than one that puts all the therapeutic eggs into the 'impairment' basket and tries to 'fix' what we usually cannot repair.

It is important to comment on how the ICF explicitly influenced the revised 2007 definition of CP (Rosenbaum et al. 2007). The new definition speaks of 'activity limitation', with the clear implication that activity is a valued aspect of child development. Nowhere are words such as 'normal' or 'typical' used or even implied. Rather, this version of the definition identifies the *impact* of the underlying impairments of body structure and function on 'activity'. This idea contrasts importantly with that developed by epidemiologists in the Western Australia Group (Blair et al. 2007). In their approach to CP for epidemiological purposes, even the presence of neurological signs (problems in body structure and function) without limitations in activity (function) is enough to qualify someone for inclusion under the label of CP. The revised CP definition uses the ICF approach, which includes an important focus on function built into its basic wording.

The ICF appears to have considerable stimulus value and seems to have caught people's attention much more widely, in a few years, than the ICIDH ever did. Thus, for example, the GMFCS (Palisano et al. 1997, 2008) explicitly refers to the ICF concepts in classifying gross motor function in people with CP, including an emphasis on 'usual performance'. We emphasize this point because among the challenges posed by thinking about 'activity' (what people can do) and 'performance' (what people actually do) is the need to recognize the nuanced but essential difference between these related ideas. To these concepts has now been added the notion of 'capability' – blending capacity with opportunity and inclination to perform the activity (Morris 2009).

Why are these ideas important? In clinical assessments we often try to elicit best abilities ('capacity') as an indication of what might be possible for that person and what we might want to focus on in treatment programmes. One need only think about how we assess the mobility of a child with CP in the clinic – removing physical obstacles, watching them move on smooth (but not slippery) surfaces, providing lots of verbal encouragement, etc. However, we may not stop to take account of whether the child actually wants (and is encouraged) to continue to do those activities that we see they have the capacity to perform during an assessment. We can too easily assume that this is what the child ought to do 'out there' on crowded, slippery or uneven surfaces – and then be disappointed by reports of a less functional 'performance' than we know to be within the child's repertoire (their best 'capacity'). We may also misinterpret a person's 'failure' to do what they are capable of achieving as evidence of a psychological or physical lapse. But of course, just because someone is capable of performing an activity does not mean that they are disposed to do it, or to do it all the time, in all environments and circumstances.

These three related but distinct concepts – capacity, performance and capability – regarding what people can and do achieve represent an important new way to think about how we evaluate children and what they actually do, and how we might be able to help them achieve their goals rather than ours. As may be apparent, these ideas about how to use the ICF in clinical practice are still evolving (Rosenbaum and Gorter 2011). Their adoption and application will, we believe, help both parents and service providers to be better able to consider the goals of interventions in the context of these ideas.

References

Blair E, Badawi N, Watson L (2007) Definition and classification of the cerebral palsies: the Australian view. *Dev Med Child Neurol* 49 (Suppl. 109): 33–4.

Boyce W, Gowland C, Rosenbaum P et al. (1995) The Gross Motor Performance Measure: validity and responsiveness of a measure of quality of movement. *Phys Ther* 75: 603–13.

Morris C (2009) Measuring participation in childhood disability: does the capability approach improve our understanding? *Dev Med Child Neurol* 51: 92–4.

Palisano RJ (2006) A collaborative model of service delivery for children with movement disorders: a framework for evidence-based decision making. *Phys Ther* 86: 1295–305.

Palisano R, Rosenbaum P, Walter S, Russell D, Wood E, Galuppi B (1997) Development and reliability of a system to classify gross motor function in children with cerebral palsy. *Dev Med Child Neurol* 39: 214–23.

Palisano RJ, Rosenbaum P, Bartlett D, Livingston MH (2008) Content validity of the Expanded and Revised Gross Motor Function Classification System. *Dev Med Child Neurol* 50: 744.

Rosenbaum P (1998) But what can you do for them? Editorial. *Dev Med Child Neurol* 40: 579.

Rosenbaum P (2007) The environment and childhood disability: opportunities to expand our horizons. Editorial. *Dev Med Child Neurol* 49: 563.

Rosenbaum PL, Gorter JW (2011) The 'F-words' in childhood disability: I swear this is how we should think! *Child Care Health Dev* doi:10.1111/j.1365–2214.2011.01338.x

Rosenbaum PL, Stewart D (2004) The WHO International Classification of Functioning, Disability and Health. A model to guide clinical thinking, practice and research in the field of cerebral palsy. *Sem Pediatr Neurol* 11: 5–10.

Rosenbaum P, Paneth N, Leviton A, Goldstein M, Bax M (2007) Definition and classification document. In: *The Definition and Classification of Cerebral Palsy*. Baxter P (ed.) *Dev Med Child Neurol* 49 (Suppl. 2): 8–14.

World Health Organization (1980) *International Classification of Impairment, Activity and Participation (ICIDH-2)*. Geneva: World Health Organization.

World Health Organization (2001) *International Classification of Functioning, Disability and Health (ICF)*. Geneva: World Health Organization.

Chapter 8

Cerebral palsy and the family

Overview

In so far as the context in which children grow up and develop is their family, it is essential to plan and execute effective connections and communication with parents of disabled children from the outset of their unexpected journey into a world they did not plan to enter. We begin with a brief consideration of the importance of how to convey 'bad news' about the diagnosis of cerebral palsy (CP) and present ideas about how to follow this up with the family and others in their circle. We then review research evidence about the impact on parental health of raising a child with a chronic condition. Family-centred service is an evidence-based approach to service provision that we believe should be an essential aspect of all the 'processes' of working with families. Finally, we outline research opportunities to move the field forward.

Traditional views of illness and disability focused on the biomedical aspects of the problem. Interventions were directed at whatever aspects of 'body structures and functions' might be influenced with the best aspects of biomedicine; in the past this was often the only preoccupation of service providers. Today, as discussed in Chapter 7, the World Health Organization's International Classification of Functioning, Disability and Health framework reminds us to expand our view and to take into account, among other factors, the 'environmental' dimensions of people's lives. For children, the essential environment is their family (Rosenbaum 2007, 2008).

It is a truism, but important to state formally, that, like all childhood conditions, CP must be considered and managed in the context of the family. Children with CP never present on their own. Their parents or others in the family's orbit (e.g. grandparents or a community physician) identify concerns about the child's development or function, and these concerns bring the child to the attention of professionals. It is therefore essential that all of what we do as service providers is carried out with an awareness of and sensitivity to the challenges faced by parents and families as they strive to understand what is happening with their young child and how best to raise their child.

This chapter addresses several linked themes about the family. We begin with a discussion of communication with parents, including the challenge of sharing 'bad news'. We then describe opportunities, with parents' permission, to engage with the wider circle of family and friends. We report on research that describes the long-term challenges to health and well-being faced by parents who are raising children with 'complicated lives'. Finally, we consider the ways that the behaviours and actions of healthcare professionals can have a positive impact on families.

Theme 1: communication with families

Telling 'bad news': the physician's first responsibility

Among the most challenging responsibilities faced by health professionals working with families of children with disabilities or other serious or chronic illnesses is the initial sharing of the 'bad news'. We believe that physicians must accept this responsibility, and that all members of the team need to be aware of what has been communicated. This is important because of the essential roles filled by developmental therapists and others in addition to doctors, and of the downstream impact on the family of this aspect of our work.

Unfortunately, at times the neonatologist or paediatrician who recognizes the likelihood that a child is at high risk of developing CP, or is in fact showing early clinical signs, does not communicate this information in an appropriate disclosure interview. They may refer the child to a physiotherapist – something that we agree is important. However, that professional is then faced with communicating with and advising a family to whom the specific issues about their child have not been explicitly articulated. The therapist is often at a significant disadvantage because they do not feel that they are in a position to give a 'diagnosis'. In fact, in many jurisdictions they may be legally prevented from doing so because making a diagnosis is a 'designated medical act' that can only be done by specific professionals. We cannot stress too strongly the importance of early referral to an expert (or at least an experienced) physician who can have an appropriate 'disclosing' interview with the parents and who will have ongoing clinical responsibility working with the family and the clinical team.

Professionals often experience the process of 'truth disclosure' as a necessary evil – one we can easily try to avoid or complete as quickly as possible because most of us feel extremely uncomfortable and want to get away. We are aware of the old idea that people want to 'shoot the messenger' – and we may fear being blamed for the child's situation. We may also be uncomfortable with the emotional responses of parents when they hear the news that their child has a permanent condition.

It is important to discuss each of these issues thoughtfully, because both experience and the literature indicate that the realities can be rather different from this bleak picture, and that effective communication can be rewarding for everyone concerned.

To begin with, it needs to be recognized that the 'telling' is not a single 'event' or discussion, but rather is a process that unfolds over time. That is to say, we need to be prepared to have several conversations with families about their child's predicament and not assume that, having been told once, they have grasped the issues and that they and we can move on. Their understanding and interpretation of their child's situation will evolve over the days and weeks after we first talk. Our capacity to clarify what has been said can also lead to a better understanding of the realities by everyone involved, including the professionals. This in turn may provide us with insights into how parental interpretations of their child's predicament are impacting on their thoughts and actions, and provide opportunities to reformulate – perhaps with other words and metaphors – what we know and foresee for that child and family.

There is, of course, a first discussion with parents when we know, or very strongly suspect, that their child has an impairment. But a brief consideration of the broader situation and context will make it apparent that the actual 'disclosure' comes at a time when the parents are already worried and concerned. They have either identified problems themselves or have agreed with the concerns of others that led to their child being assessed in the first place. After all, they are in the clinic allowing their child to be evaluated. They are therefore primed in some way, and often have worries about issues that are even more serious than the condition we are about to discuss. In other words, whatever we have to say is not a bolt from the blue, but more a specific articulation of what they already either know or fear.

In the days of universally available information (especially through the Internet) and a public that is increasingly well informed, many parents have already worked out what their child's problems are. Why, then, do they come to us at all?

We believe that they want confirmation, clarification, perspectives, advice and the benefit of our experience, but they are seldom completely unaware of what might be happening. In fact it is often useful first to ask parents about their worst fears regarding what we are about to discuss. That way our conversation can be rooted at least in part in our awareness of those concerns, allowing us to confirm or to clarify what they are thinking.

Several elements of the disclosure interview and process are clearly and consistently identified in the literature (e.g. Cunningham et al. 1984). Parents want to be told as soon as we know. They want to be told together, in private. They want the truth, but in language that is understandable to them. They want to be left with hope, and they want control over the pace of the telling (Cassel 1982). There is a profound difference between telling the truth at a pace that the family can absorb (which we believe should always be done) and telling 'the truth, the whole truth and everything we know' all at once, as if we were discussing CP with students in the clinic and feel a need to disgorge all the facts.

It is worth noting briefly the idea that the same words, asking what might seem to be a straightforward and appropriate questions (e.g. 'What is CP?'), take on completely different meanings depending on the context of the question. Consider how we might have a conversation with parents who have just been told about their child's diagnosis and contrast that with how we might respond from an academic perspective to the students and trainees when they ask us about CP. Answers to parents should always be specific to their child's strengths and issues – what Seigler (1975) calls 'prognostication' – while a conversation with learners is likely to be far more wide-ranging about the condition than about 'this child with these manifestations of the condition'.

The challenges of this kind of communication include how to pace the presentation of information. If we overwhelm people with too much information when their guard may be down and when they may be unable to deal with a tidal wave of detail, we risk missing the chance to communicate effectively and drowning them with information. Thus, giving parents control of the interview is an essential dimension of the process.

At the end of the initial interview it can be helpful to enquire of the parents who will be telephoning them when they get home to ask about today's visit. We then ask parents to tell us what they will say to those people (often, for example, worried grandparents). If the answer is 'We will tell them what you have said', we push them, perhaps with some role play, to use their own words to explain things as if they were on the telephone responding to others' questions. This can be a very useful way to learn how the parents have heard and interpreted our conversation, and can afford an immediate opportunity to correct what might be any major misconceptions.

Experience and the literature would suggest that parents vividly remember the first telling, especially the emotional tenor of the event, even years later. They recall good experiences (when the 'telling' was well paced, sensitive and responsive to their needs) and especially the unpleasant encounters with people they judge to have been insensitive, brusque or patronizing. It is our belief that this initial impression matters greatly, in so far as it may condition whether people subsequently trust professionals and our advice or are wary of us – and by extension the whole system – because of what they consider to have been less than caring communication from us.

Where else do parents get their information? Asking parents directly about what they are hearing and reading easily opens the conversation. They read books, listen to other parents of disabled children and receive advice from almost everyone. Of course, in today's world the Internet is an instant, powerful and pervasive repository of ideas that range from very useful and credible contemporary sources of information to sites that are nothing more than advertisements for unproven miracle cures, replete with testimonials. In addition, none of the available sites is discussing this specific child and family. This can put parents in the unenviable position of having to weigh what may be conflicting ideas about everything from causal factors in CP to recommendations for treatments and therapy programmes that promise far more than many of us are currently able to deliver. Some of these issues have been discussed in the context of 'alternative' treatments (Rosenbaum 1997, 2003; Rosenbaum and Stewart 2002), but the basic ideas are relevant to all information to which parents are exposed. These issues are also discussed in Chapter 11.

Telling 'bad news': the follow-up
Over the years, one experience that has been both helpful and fascinating is to meet again with the family within a few days of the initial disclosure and to go over the issues once more. We also offer parents the opportunity to bring with them to this second visit anyone they think should hear the story 'from the horse's mouth'. This usually has included grandparents, close friends, the nanny, aunts, uncles, the family doctor – whoever is important to the parents and who they feel should be there. Several aspects of this process should be highlighted.

First, when we meet for the second time we ask the parents to tell us, in their own words, how they now understand their child's situation and how they are explaining it to others. We listen for their understanding of aetiology, functional prognosis, interventions that might be available – whatever they report back can help reveal how they are processing and interpreting the 'facts' of their family's dilemma.

This conversation provides an opportunity once again to hear their interpretation of the information we have tried to provide in the previous meeting. We listen for what might be misunderstandings, and for possible gaps in the story that can be filled in this time. We ask what they have heard/read/discovered since the previous meeting, because invariably parents and their families have done their own research and often have a myriad of questions based on these discoveries. Whether and how this new information applies to their particular child can be helpful both in the specific detail it provides and more broadly to help people understand that specific facts about causation or treatment of CP may be relevant in some situations but not in others. We consider that this kind of open discussion helps parents to develop a trusting relationship with us – something we believe will be important as they work with us and the systems we represent.

A second aspect of this kind of meeting is that it provides an opportunity for the people parents trust most, such as their own parents or siblings, to ask the questions they themselves might fear to ask. On many occasions we have seen Uncle Charlie or Aunt Rose act as the Greek chorus, becoming the spokesperson for the family on the parents' behalf. On the assumption that this arrangement meets the family's needs (given that these people have been invited to this discussion), it affords an opportunity to discuss a host of issues that might have been raised in private family discussions that preceded this meeting. These issues can range from the likelihood of another child being born with CP (either to the parents or in the extended family) to questions about the latest interventions, be they conventional or alternative and complementary. The fact that everyone who attends is exposed to the same ideas at the same time makes it more likely that as a group they will hear, understand and recall the discussions later on.

Third, we need to be aware of the 'generational sandwich' in which many parents find themselves. It is thus important to highlight the particular roles and potential contributions of grandparents. As developmentalists, the people with whom we work are the parents of the children and young people with CP. We know them in their roles as parents and fellow adults. It may be easy to forget that these parents are almost always someone's 'child', and that they may be treated that way by the child with CP's grandparents. After all, as parents themselves, the grandparents are also worried about their (adult) child's predicament. Thus, for example, in their efforts to be supportive to and protective of their 'child', the grandparents may seek to downplay the seriousness of what the parents have heard from us. This can put the parents in an invidious position of having to credit (or discredit) one source of information and support over another.

Being a generation older, the grandparents might have what today would be considered as 'old-fashioned' ideas about CP or disability. They may need help to gain a 'modern' understanding of these issues. If they have known of someone with CP in an earlier era (e.g. a schoolmate, a family member, a friend's child, someone in the community), their experience can range from very negative to very positive. Whatever the case, that specific experience needs to be identified and incorporated into the discussions, because it will be looming in the shadows and will probably inflect discussions within the family at some point.

On the other hand, of course, grandparents often have resources of time and money as well as perspective, wisdom and life experience that can be invaluable to the young parents, who are our primary concern. Being able to involve grandparents in their grandchild's orbit – only, of course, with parents' permission – may provide the young parents embarking on this complex journey with added layers of support.

It will be obvious that any time that a meeting with the whole family is possible such an opportunity reflects the availability of the extended network and the parents' capacity to mobilize resources that are likely to be helpful to both their child and themselves. It also offers them a buffer between their own family's worries and concerns and what we hope is the security that a good relationship with caring professionals can provide. Note that this is but one of many illustrations of how one can take a strengths-based approach to our work, striving to have the family identify and build on their child's and family's strengths and resources as the foundation of whatever they do.

Theme 2: the impact of disability on parental health and well-being

A relatively unrecognized aspect of 'CP and the family' concerns the accumulating evidence of the impact of childhood disability (including but not limited to CP) on the physical and mental health of parents (Brehaut et al. 2004, 2009; Lach et al. 2009). Whether one uses findings from clinical studies (Brehaut et al. 2004) or data from population-based surveys (Brehaut et al. 2009; Lach et al. 2009), there is robust evidence that parenting children with early-onset chronic conditions and disabilities, including CP, is strongly and consistently associated with a considerable impact on the well-being of the parents of these children.

It would be tempting to argue that the probable causal direction of this relationship is that parental ill health leads to an increased risk of developmental problems in their children. Indeed, in some developmental disability situations this may be the case, in so far as many health problems and disabilities are inversely related to socioeconomic status. In addition, there are gradients of impact of sociodemographic disadvantage on the health and developmental outcomes of children. It is therefore easy to assume that parental health problems 'cause' childhood disabilities.

Of course, an equally plausible interpretation is that these issues co-vary in relation to a common third factor, namely 'socioeconomic disadvantage', by whatever mechanisms this factor might operate. (See also Chapters 4 and 6, where issues of causation are discussed.)

From what is currently understood about putative causal pathways in the genesis of CP (Stanley et al. 2000), it is unlikely that parental health problems 'cause' CP. However, even if it were the case that parental disadvantage were a contributing factor in the emergence of conditions such as CP, it seems highly likely that raising a child with a long-term challenge of health or development also creates stresses that take their toll on parental health over time. This in turn will obviously have an important impact on the child's development and well-being.

The reason for identifying these issues explicitly is that, like other neurodevelopmental conditions, CP has traditionally been considered to be a 'children's' issue. We believe that it is imperative to broaden the perspective in our work in childhood disability to recognize the roles of parents and the impact on them of raising a child who faces ongoing challenges. We like to think of a 'child-in-family' approach to the challenges associated with CP and other neurodevelopmental conditions. It then becomes appropriate to widen the scope of practice and to value our interest in the well-being of parents, being attentive to the needs of families as part of how we can best help children.

This aspect of childhood neurodisability is an area of practice that has received relatively little formal attention. Hence, not a lot is known about the causal pathways by which the stresses associated with children's disabilities might contribute to problems in parental well-being. This is an area ripe for thoughtful prospective longitudinal research to explore both the mechanisms by which chronic stress impacts on people and the potential preventability of many of these stresses.

There is a certain amount of 'received wisdom' about family dysfunction among families raising children with complicated lives. (These are illustrations of what we like to call the 'Everyone knows . . .' ideas.) For example, it is often believed that families of disabled children have a higher rate of marital failure than other families.

The findings from the literature suggest a trend but are far from conclusive. When our group explored the issues 25 years ago, we could find no consistent evidence to support this notion (Cadman et al. 1987). In a large population-based study of the health of Canadian caregivers (Brehaut et al. 2009), there were no differences in measures of marital satisfaction among parents of children with chronic health conditions compared with those with typically developing children. Similarly, when Lundeby and

Tøssebro (2008) explored Norwegian data from over 2600 families, they found that the family structure in families raising a child with a disability was similar to that of other families. Seltzer et al. (2001) also reported no difference in marital status among parents of children with a range of developmental or behavioural issues compared with a normative sample. On the other hand, a recent study by Hartley et al. (2010) on families of children with autism spectrum disorders reported a significantly higher rate of marital breakdown in index families than in a matched comparison group.

Not surprisingly it has been shown that the strength of the marital relationship is important to parental well-being (Kersh et al. 2006). This kind of observation supports the importance of an approach to service delivery that includes family well-being, as outlined in the next section of the chapter.

Theme 3: 'processes' of care – family-centred service

In the context of CP and other neurodisabilities affecting the family, we believe there is an imperative to provide services in a family-centred manner (Rosenbaum et al. 1998).

> Family-centred service is made up of a set of values, attitudes, and approaches to services for children with special needs and their families. Family-centred service recognizes that each family is unique; that the family is the constant in the child's life; and that they are the experts on the child's abilities and needs. The family works with service providers to make informed decisions about the services and supports the child and family receive. In family-centred service, the strengths and needs of all family members are considered.
>
> *CanChild* (2003a)

The reason for introducing these ideas is to provide a rationale for the importance of communication and relationship building with families. In many respects parents are as much our 'patients' as their young child. It is with them that our initial connections are made and our communication takes place. They are the child's advocates and the decision-makers to whom we must provide the best available information and perspectives, and whose questions we must answer to the best of our ability. Thus, the nature and quality of the relationships we develop with them over time matter greatly.

By engaging in partnerships with families, we empower them to be the directors of their child's lives. We then respond to the issues they identify as important to their concerns about their child and their family. One clinical example of the impact and success of an approach that respects parents' (and children's) decision-making was illustrated in an excellent study by Ketelaar and her colleagues (2001). Their randomized clinical trial demonstrated that when therapy services are directed at addressing goals set by parents and children rather than by professionals, the outcomes are measurably better and are achieved with less intervention.

It is possible to measure parents' experiences of how family-centred the services are (King et al. 1996). This work was begun in an effort to explore whether family-centred services actually matter. Cross-sectional observational research has linked 'processes' of service delivery to 'outcomes' of parental satisfaction or stress with services with parental mental health (King et al. 1999). The research, replicated in other countries (e.g. Siebes et al. 2007a,b), provides evidence that the ways in which services are experienced by parents (i.e. the extent to which they are perceived to be family-centred) can have a clear relationship with parental well-being.

There is evidence that better satisfaction is associated with better adherence to treatment recommendations. Logically, then, the processes of service delivery are very likely to impact on the extent to which families trust, respect and follow our advice. There are freely available guidelines about how to provide services that are family-centred in process and content (*CanChild* 2003b), so this approach to services should be easy to implement.

Theme 4: an issue for future research

Finally, it is worth considering an idea about which there is, to our knowledge, no solid research evidence yet available, but which may be very important as a launching pad for parents in their understanding of their child's situation. We believe that the way in which we formulate our ideas about a child's CP may be formative in how parents view their child, their child's condition, their roles as parents and their power and control to effect change in their child's life.

If, on the one hand, we present CP as a condition due to a permanent manifestation of 'brain damage' about which we can do nothing curative, we may easily convey the impression that their child is irrevocably broken or damaged and cannot be 'fixed'. The brain will never be 'normal', and until stem cells or other futuristic treatments are shown to be effective there is little to be done from a medical perspective. While this might be literally true – at least with respect to the biomedical realities of the early twenty-first century, because we cannot (yet) replace the damaged parts of the brain – the message that might be heard could lead parents to a sense of hopelessness about their child.

On the other hand, we believe that we must always convey to parents that their child with CP is first and foremost a child – and that it is the nature of children to grow, to develop, to change, to learn, to 'become'. We have argued (Rosenbaum 2009) that we need to remember that 'developmental' disabilities are conditions that do, or are likely to, affect the trajectory of a child's development, and we should do everything we can to help parents promote their child's development even when the child's biological systems work differently because of impairments. This means being less preoccupied with what is thought to be 'normal' – an idea which, in any case, we find unhelpful and often limiting.

Rather, we need to help parents keep their eye on the longer-term goal of promoting their child's emergence as a capable, confident, independent person to the best extent possible, even if the way in which the young person does things is different from the range of ways that things usually happen in typical development. It is our experience that parents can understand these ideas, and with help and support can parent their disabled child with these ideas in mind.

We want parents to be able to identify their child's abilities and to be aware of the temperamental, developmental and other capacities that make that child unique. We often start any conversation with parents by asking them what they want to brag about. This may take some parents by surprise, but they are rarely short of answers. This approach also signals to parents that we expect them to have opportunities for joy and pride in their child and not just to assume that things are always 'broken'. A careful research-based exploration of this way of communicating with parents would undoubtedly be very rewarding intellectually, and be well received by families.

References

Brehaut J, Kohen D, Raina P et al. (2004) The health of parents of children with cerebral palsy: how does it compare to other Canadian adults? *Pediatrics* 114: e182–91.

Brehaut JC, Kohen DE, Garner RE et al. (2009) Health among caregivers of children with health problems: findings from a Canadian population-based study. *Am J Public Health* 99: 1254–62.

Cadman D, Rosenbaum P, Pettingill P (1987) Prevention of emotional, behavioral, and family problems of children with chronic medical illness. *J Prev Psychiatry* 3: 147–65.

CanChild (2003a) http://www.canchild.ca/en/childrenfamilies/resources/FCSSheet1.pdf (accessed 4 January 2011).

CanChild (2003b) Available at: http://www.canchild.ca/en/childrenfamilies/fcs_sheet.asp (accessed 26 November 2010).

Cassel EJ (1982) The nature of suffering and the goals of medicine. *N Engl J Med* 306: 639–45.

Cunningham CC, Morgan PA, McGucken RB (1984) Down's syndrome: is dissatisfaction with disclosure of diagnosis inevitable? *Dev Med Child Neurol* 26: 33–9.

Hartley SL, Barker ET, Seltzer MM, Floyd F, Greenberg J, Orsmond G, Bolt D (2010) The relative risk and timing of divorce in families of children with an autism spectrum disorder. *J Family Psychol* 24: 449–57.

Kersh J, Hedvat TT, Hauser-Cram P, Warfield ME (2006) The contribution of marital quality to the well-being of parents of children with developmental disabilities. *J Intellect Disabil Res* 50: 883–93.

Ketelaar M, Vermeer A, Hart H et al. (2001) Effects of a functional therapy program on motor abilities of children with CP. *Phys Ther* 81: 1534–45.

King G, King S, Rosenbaum P, Goffin R (1999) Family-centred caregiving and well-being of parents of children with disabilities: Linking process with outcome. *J Pediatr Psychol* 24: 41–52.

King S, Rosenbaum P, King G (1996) Parents' perceptions of care-giving: development and validation of a process measure. *Dev Med Child Neurol* 38: 757–72.

Lach LM, Kohen DE, Garner RE (2009) The health and psychosocial functioning of caregivers of children with neurodevelopmental disorders. *Disabil Rehabil* 31: 741–52.

Lundeby H, Tøssebro J (2008) Family structure in Norwegian families of children with disabilities. *J Appl Res Intellect Disabil* 21: 246–56.

Rosenbaum PL (1997) 'Alternative' treatments for children with disabilities: thoughts from the trenches. *Paediatr Child Health* 2: 122–4.

Rosenbaum PL (2003) Controversial treatment of spasticity: exploring alternative therapies for motor function in children with cerebral palsy. *J Child Neurol* 18: S89–94.

Rosenbaum P (2007) The environment and childhood disability: opportunities to expand our horizons. Editorial. *Dev Med Child Neurol* 49: 563.

Rosenbaum P (2008) Families of children with chronic conditions: opportunities to widen the scope of pediatric practice. *J Pediatr* 153: 304–5.

Rosenbaum P (2009) Putting child development back into developmental disabilities. *Dev Med Child Neurol* 51: 251.

Rosenbaum P, Stewart D (2002) Alternative and complementary therapies for children and youth with disabilities. *Infants Young Child* 15: 51–9.

Rosenbaum P, King S, Law M, King G, Evans J (1998) Family-centred services: a conceptual framework and research review. *Phys Occup Ther Pediatr* 18: 1–20.

Seltzer MM, Greenberg JS, Floyd FJ, Pettee Y, Hong J (2001) Life course impacts of parenting a child with a disability. *Am J Mental Retardation* 106: 265–86.

Siebes RC, Maassen GH, Wijnroks L et al. (2007a) Quality of paediatric rehabilitation from the parent perspective: validation of the short Measure of Processes of Care (MPOC-20) in the Netherlands. *Clin Rehabil* 21: 62–72.

Siebes RC, Wijnroks L, Ketelaar M, van Schie PE, Gorter JW, Vermeer A (2007b) Parent participation in paediatric rehabilitation treatment centres in the Netherlands: a parents' viewpoint. *Child Care Health Dev* 33: 196–205.

Siegler M (1975) Pascal's wager and the hanging of crepe. *N Engl J Med* 293: 853–7.

Stanley F, Blair, E, Alberman E (2000) *Cerebral Palsies: Epidemiology and Causal Pathways*. Clinics in Developmental Medicine No. 151. London: Mac Keith Press.

Part 3

Clinical perspectives in cerebral palsy

Chapter 9

Clinical recognition, diagnosis and assessment of children with cerebral palsy

---

Overview

In this chapter, we first discuss the range of presentations of cerebral palsy (CP) that can be reported by families. There will be times when there have been no identified antenatal and/or neonatal factors that are known to have the potential to compromise development. At other times the suspicion about a child's risk of developing CP will be relatively high. In either case it is important to obtain a systematic review of the mother's biomedical background and the child's early history. The assessment of the child should address both issues of general development and a systematic neurological and functional evaluation. Thereafter we amplify the details of the additional investigations and examinations that may need to be undertaken. Finally we outline the range of actions that should be taken once the consultation process has been completed to support the family towards a comprehensive management plan.

Suspicion about the possibility that a child has CP is often based on a history of adverse antenatal or perinatal events. When no such concerns or issues are communicated to parents by professionals in the early days of an infant's development, recognition of the likelihood or even the possibility that a child may have a developmental disability usually emerges from parental or family observations.

From a professional's perspective, we need to consider the questions 'What did this infant or child "look like" before the formal diagnosis of CP was made?' and 'What were the early signs that led parents to be concerned about their child's motor development?'

It is again appropriate to emphasize that while our primary focus is on CP, both the principles and much of the detail of this chapter can be applied equally to other neuro-developmental disabilities.

Presentation following parental concerns

In the majority of cases, children with CP present with some 'deficit' in their early development. Parents note that their child is having difficulty in reaching motor milestones that they know to be part of typical development. Their observations may be based on their own experience with previous children, comparison with the children of friends and family or comments from concerned relatives. They may comment on their child feeling 'stiff' or perhaps 'floppy', or they may note asymmetries of function. Whether they have had other children or have read books on child development, parents will generally have an idea about when infants typically achieve skills such as head and trunk control, sitting, rolling, creeping and crawling, pulling to stand and walking.

Parents' interpretations of their child's apparent difficulties can vary considerably, depending in part on individual circumstances. If, for example, the child was born preterm, they may already anticipate problems with the child's development based on the perinatal and neonatal course and on things that were said in response to parents' questions in the neonatal intensive care unit about how 'these babies' develop (Rosenbaum 2006a). They may also forget that we adjust ('correct') for the amount of an infant's prematurity. This allows us to assess development in terms of postconceptional rather than 'birthday' age. If the child is a twin or triplet, parents may, on the one hand, make excuses for a child with motor difficulties or, on the other hand, expect that whichever infant is developing fastest is the 'normal' one and that others must be 'delayed'. In the latter situation, the task of professionals is to sort out variation from 'abnormality', a task that may require repeated observations over time (Rosenbaum 2006b).

Occasionally the presentation of a child's difficulties may be subtler. Not only may parents not worry about differences in motor development, but also they may be proud of what they perceive to be evidence of advanced motor skills. They may interpret their daughter's lower limb extensor tone and toe standing – signs that are usually indications of upper motor neurone difficulties often associated with spastic CP – as early evidence of a possible career in ballet. They might comment on how 'strong' their infant with extensor tone is, misinterpreting spasticity for motor precocity. They may be pleased that their young child is going to be left handed like a parent or grandparent, again misinterpreting early signs of a hemisyndrome as indications of advanced motor skills. We must therefore listen attentively to parents who describe what appear to be signs of gross or fine motor precocity, and consider carefully both the motor behaviours and the interpretation of what the child demonstrates on assessment in order to decide whether there is a problem.

As is further detailed below, it is also important to consider this variety of possible presentations within a number of contexts. These include how the child is perceived to be developing as a whole, and also whether there are relevant family and social circumstances that might influence the interpretation of clinical findings.

Standardized 'screening' examinations

It is only after a child is born that any form of detailed neurological evaluation can be undertaken. Debate continues as to whether all newborn infants should undergo detailed neurological examinations ('screening' everyone for CP) or whether this should be confined to those in whom there is concern that there may be abnormalities of neurological functioning.

For several reasons the authors have considerable doubt that a universal screening process for CP should be undertaken at a community level (Al-Qabandi et al. 2011). First, we know of no proven sensitive and specific screening tools that have been well developed and studied for this purpose. Second, there is a considerable potential negative impact on families whose children are subject to 'false-positive' and 'false-negative' tests. Third, early child development shows considerable variability, and, other than in the most apparent situations of 'severe' impairment, it is often difficult to interpret the clinical meaning of early 'signs' of neurological development. Fourth, unlike screening for phenylketonuria or congenital hypothyroidism – the classic screening paradigms on which others are often modelled – there are no proven specific 'treatments' for infants and young children with CP. In fact, in many communities there are often long waiting times to access appropriate developmental services. For these reasons we recommend, in addition to thoughtful assessment of all infants at well-baby visits, careful surveillance of children known to be at increased risk of neurodevelopmental challenges (described below) as well as case finding in these special populations.

It is of interest that available methods for examination vary from what is termed 'the classical neurological examination of young infants' (the predictive value of which is uncertain) to observational methods such as the general movement assessment approach of Precht and his colleagues (Einspieler et al. 2005), which appear to be more useful as indicators of later developmental challenges. However, a correlation between abnormal findings and later demonstration of CP does not appear to have been established on a population basis. At a minimum, however, all newborn infants require a general paediatric examination that includes an accurate measurement of the head circumference.

More detailed examinations do need to be undertaken in infants who have been born significantly preterm, in those who are thought to be at risk of neurological abnormalities for whatever reason, in those who present with abnormal neurological features including seizures and in those with dysmorphic features.

What is very important in population studies is that there must be an opportunity for follow-up. There also need to be robust assessment processes and the correlation of any investigation results with the emerging clinical picture of the child's function (Rosenbaum et al. 2009). For a detailed review of this subject, reference should be made to the useful text of Cioni and Mercuri (2008).

The clinical history: maternal and infant features

What do paediatricians and neurologists look for when CP is a possibility? The first element of assessment is, of course, always the child's history. It is important to elicit a history of maternal and family factors such as maternal health problems (e.g. diabetes or previous pregnancy losses) that might suggest a predisposition to problems in maintaining healthy pregnancies. The infant's 'developmental' history as a fetus can be helpful with respect to an account of intrauterine movement, such as changes in patterns at a specific time in the pregnancy that might constitute evidence of a maternal or pregnancy-related problem.

Obvious factors such as preterm and multiple births (including the loss of a twin in pregnancy) will increase the threshold for suspicion about the possibility that a current problem in infant development is 'CP' and is related to (perhaps even 'caused by') these aspects of a child's history (see also Chapter 3, where issues of causation are discussed). In addition, of course, the parents' reports of their child's function described above will provide hints about the possibility of developmental problems, as will concerns identified by grandparents and others whom the parents trust.

Whether infants were born at term or preterm, their condition at birth requires review. Basic data such as birthweight and head size, related to appropriate norms, need to be evaluated, as does their neonatal presentation. Was there evidence of cardiorespiratory depression at birth with low Apgar scores and evidence of acidosis? Did the infant require admission to a neonatal intensive care unit? Was there evidence of a neonatal encephalopathy with seizures? Were there difficulties in establishing oral feeding? Was there significant jaundice or evidence of neonatal sepsis? Were neurological investigations undertaken, including electroencephalography and imaging studies, and if so what did they show? These issues are comprehensively reviewed in a variety of texts (see, for example, Rennie et al. [2008] and Levene and Chervenak [2009], to which reference should be made for further detail).

The history then needs to be brought up to date by obtaining information from parents or carers with respect to the child's current abilities. These consist of gross motor, fine motor and oromotor function, as well as vision, hearing, language, cognitive functioning, behaviour and social skills. We find it helpful to have a checklist or proforma in order to ensure that all important information is elicited and recorded. Clearly the data obtained then require to be correlated with those obtained from the clinical examination, as is detailed in the following section.

Clinical examination of the child with cerebral palsy

General assessment

Descriptions of how best to engage children, and their parents or carers, in the consultation and examination are outside the remit of this chapter. So also are detailed descriptions of the general and neurological examinations of children. For all of these issues, reference should be made to a variety of standard texts such as that of Forfar and Arneil (McIntosh et al. 2008).

Rather, in this section we focus on the key points to consider, record and evaluate when examining children who are referred as possibly having CP or another neurological disability. We should also make clear that we are referring principally to the medical examination and that in no way does this replace appropriate standardized and other specific targeted clinical assessments undertaken by psychologists and therapists.

For the paediatric examiner, a useful test of how complex and detailed the assessment needs to be is to ask the question 'Will the information that has been obtained be sufficient to write an informed explanatory note to the family or a helpful referral letter to a professional colleague?'

We first emphasize the need to be opportunistic in the observations that are made even though the formal recording of these findings has to be rigorously systematic. In fact, much of the assessment of motor function – postural control, arm and hand function, and lower extremity activity – can be observed during the course of the history taking. If the chance to examine lower limb joint ranges comes early in the assessment, then it has to be taken as it may not recur without the need to cause distress. We tend to leave head circumference measurement to the end, and the addition of feathers to a tape measure to make it into a head dress has an appeal to older children in the UK.

The issue of taking and using photographs and videos in clinical assessment requires thought. It goes without saying that fully informed consent is required. The problem is that the original consent form for photographs in a generic clinical record that will be used by the original clinicians cannot automatically be translated to later users without a separate consent. The latter should of course also include the child. Hence, we recommend the practice of using photographs and video only exceptionally, and for specific and time-limited purposes. These days parents increasingly bring home videos with them to clinic, and certainly can be asked to do so if there are specific aspects of behaviour or function that are best captured outside a clinic visit.

What are the essential elements of the assessment? General presentation comes first on the list. Is the child alert and responsive? Is their social interaction developmentally appropriate?

Should dysmorphic features be considered to be present, they require careful evaluation within the context of how other family members may look. It is here that review of family photographs and earlier photographs of the child can be helpful (perhaps by asking the family to bring in their 'baby book').

At some stage that requires clinical judgement, the child needs to be undressed, at least down to the underclothes. Weight, height (or length) and head size should be serially recorded and charted systematically in all children. We recommend using the charts published by Day et al. (2012) that compare weight for different degrees of severity of CP (see Appendix IV), which should be available and referred to as part of clinical follow-up.

Neurological assessment
A formal neurological examination in children should always be undertaken as an essential component of the clinical examination, although the degree of detail may vary depending on factors such as cooperation and opportunity.

Within this context, it is helpful to observe and comment on a child's posture and postural control, both at rest and when active, the ranges of joint movement and the presence of any contractures and deformities including the presence of any abnormal spinal curvature. Overt asymmetries must be noted. If present, these may be a consequence of impaired growth or impaired function or both, especially in children with hemiplegic presentations. It is also necessary to note the presence and distribution of any involuntary movements and whether or not there is evidence of impaired coordination affecting gross motor, fine motor or oromotor functioning.

Wherever possible, there should be an assessment of muscle tone. We must keep in mind that this part of the clinical examination is being used to determine whether the affected child has significant corticospinal tract (pyramidal tract) or significant extrapyramidal tract motor abnormalities or indeed impairment of cerebellar functioning. Muscle tone assessment can be particularly challenging as definitions and understanding of the concepts of spasticity, dystonia and hypotonia, the three common muscle tone abnormalities that are seen in CP, vary across authorities and clinicians (see Sanger et al. 2003, 2010). We find that the most clinically applicable definition of spasticity is that it is an increase in velocity-dependent muscle tone in response to stretching relaxed muscle. The most useful way to think of dystonia within the context of CP is that there are involuntary fluctuations of muscle tone. In addition, it is also important to attempt to evaluate whether there is muscle weakness and to distinguish this from hypotonia (reduced muscle tone). As discussed in Chapter 4, we recommend the use of the Surveillance of Cerebral Palsy in Europe group approach to the characterization of motor impairments (Cans 2000).

Functional assessment
It is next appropriate to consider gross motor function from both the history provided and examination. Within the context of always assigning a Gross Motor Function Classification System (GMFCS) level, it may be helpful to have a copy of the Expanded and Revised GMFCS (Palisano et al. 2008) available as a desktop tool (this is available for free at http://www.canchild.ca/en/measures/gmfcs_expanded_revised.asp and is reproduced in Appendix I). Specific note needs to be taken of the head posture and the degree of head control that is present, whether or not the child can sit independently or needs support for sitting and whether or not there is any independent mobility by rolling, scooting (on the back) or crawling. It is also useful to note whether the child can undertake transfers, and if so with what degree of assistance.

For children with greater motor ability, we need to ascertain whether they walk independently and ,if so, from what age. Observation of gait is then important with reference to factors such as asymmetry, other abnormalities of posture and the pattern and speed of walking. It is also often helpful to note the child's ability on stairs, in standing on either foot and in hopping. For a more detailed description of gait evaluation and its range of possible abnormalities, reference should be made to Morris and Dias (2007) and Gage et al. (2009).

So far as upper limb function is concerned, it is helpful to make use of the Manual Ability Classification System (Eliasson et al. 2006), which is available for free at www. macs.nu and provided in Appendix II. This system is not yet as well established as the GMFCS but does provide a useful summary of manual function. Superimposed on this it is then helpful to detail hand preference, with a description of any difficulties in play activities, in undertaking writing or keyboard work and in daily living activities, for example in fastening buttons or zips and in feeding skills.

In appropriate circumstances, getting a child to draw a figure offers useful information not only concerning fine motor skills but also with respect to a range of perceptual and cognitive abilities.

The assessment of oromotor function has a number of components. The first is the child's chewing and swallowing abilities. Where there is any concern about these, and particularly if there is concern about whether swallowing is safe, then relevant specialist assessments and investigations are mandatory, often performed by a specialized feeding team. As part of this assessment it is important to enquire about drooling, especially as helpful interventions may be possible.

The second component of oromotor function that it is necessary to evaluate is speech. Intelligibility, quality and clarity of speech sound production should be noted.

Visual and ophthalmological assessments are next required. It is important always to ask 'How well does your child see?' Visual impairment is easily missed and specific examination of a child's ability to fix, follow and use vision is required. Note is required about whether a strabismus or nystagmus is present.

Although hearing impairment is uncommon in CP (with the exception of that caused by kernicterus), a child's hearing also requires assessment via parental history as well as expert audiological evaluation.

Sequentially, an assessment of language comprehension and whether this is age appropriate is next undertaken. Here it is often helpful to record examples of what has been seen during the consultation or reported by the parents. It is particularly common for ability in this area of functioning to be overestimated, especially when a child relies on eye pointing or other non-verbal forms of communication. Note as well that parents almost always report – accurately – 'Our child understands everything we say to him'. What they (and we) may fail to recognize is that adults automatically tailor their communication to the child's comprehension level. Thus, unless a formal assessment is done, a child's limitations in receptive language capacity may go unrecognized.

Similar considerations apply to the clinical evaluation of the cognitive abilities of children with CP; here again, although an experienced clinician can obtain an impression, this always requires confirmation by appropriate psychological testing. This is discussed further below.

Are investigations required?

Conventionally, the next steps following recognition that a child has CP are to consider appropriate investigations, to arrange for relevant and comprehensive multidisciplinary assessments and to refer for consideration of appropriate interventions. All of these activities overlap with one other, with the ongoing processes of communicating with families, and with parental adaptation.

In part this process will depend on how secure the clinical diagnosis of CP is. For example, in the absence of a relevant perinatal history, it is necessary to consider carefully whether the child's underlying brain abnormality is indeed static or whether it may be progressive. If there is any clinical suggestion of the latter, then relevant investigations are required. The extent and nature of these will be determined by the clinical presentation, and King and Stephenson (2009) provide a useful guide.

Other investigations may be determined by the nature of the clinical presentation even when the diagnosis of CP is secure. For example, electroencephalography studies will be relevant if there is a history or the clinical likelihood of seizures.

There are mixed views about whether routine magnetic resonance brain imaging should be part of the investigation protocol for children who are considered to have CP. This is advocated by some authorities (Russman and Ashwal 2004); whether or not this investigation is undertaken would appear to depend as much on available resources as on the merits or otherwise of the knowledge that can be derived from this procedure. In our experience, parents vary in their wish to obtain radiological confirmation of the extent and pattern of brain damage, especially if this is not going to alter either the diagnosis or the management.

It is also fair to say that in spite of there being increasingly fast magnetic resonance imaging techniques, the need for many children to undergo general anaesthesia for magnetic resonance imaging is a point that weighs heavily with many parents and indeed many professionals.

Against this background, it is the authors' practice to always offer magnetic resonance brain imaging as part of their diagnostic evaluation.

Interpretation of the clinical findings

It has been pointed out elsewhere (Rosenbaum 2006a) that we must always be aware of the challenge of interpreting the evidence from history and assessment. The most obvious cautions come with respect to elements of the child's history. Just because a child was born early or was a member of a multiple pregnancy (predisposing them epidemiologically to an increased risk of CP) does not automatically mean that their motor development differences are evidence of CP. In fact, unless one makes allowance for preterm birth and 'corrects' the infant's age accordingly, it is all too easy to misinterpret what seems to be 'delay' as 'abnormality' (Rosenbaum 2006b).

It can at times be very challenging to decide on a first assessment whether a 'difference' constitutes an 'abnormality'. Under these circumstances it is often reasonable to delay making a definitive diagnosis and to reassess the infant or young child within a matter of weeks or months, explicitly choosing a time that is typically associated with a high probability that specific motor skills should have appeared developmentally.

For example, if we see a 4-month-old with apparent lag in head and trunk control on pulling to sitting, and are uncertain whether the 'delay' is 'abnormal', it is appropriate to reassess the child at 6 months developmental age or a bit later, when both head and trunk control are usually well consolidated and most infants are able to maintain head and trunk posture with (and at times without) lower trunk support from an adult. One might think of this manoeuvre as a 'test of time'. Persistence of postural difficulties at 6 months considerably increases our concern about the significance of problems in motor development, whereas improvements may provide all the reassurance we need, or at least allow us to continue follow-up without labelling the pattern of motor development with a 'diagnosis'. In terms used in the literature discussing the critical appraisal of evidence, one might be experiencing a fair degree of uncertainty about the diagnosis at 4 months; the 'pretest probability' of CP may be moderately high. (If we are already very worried, or very reassured, about a child's development then this is not an issue – it is the uncertainty in between that is problematic.) If at 6 months the child has made good developmental motor progress, the 'post-test probability' of CP is much reduced; on the other hand, continuing functional difficulties make the 'post-test probability' of CP much higher.

Particular care is required when examining infants who have been born very preterm. Under these circumstances there is a wider range of normal responses than in children born at term (see the discussion by Mercuri et al. in Cioni and Mercuri 2008).

When assessing a child, it may be useful to think about both the 'quantity' and 'quality' of motor performance (Rosenbaum 2006a). Milestones are classically used to describe the quantity of development. They indicate whether a child has reached a specific 'marker' thought to be typical for children of that age. In themselves, however, milestones tell us little about the 'quality' of the performance any more than the milestone indicators on a road tell us anything about the nature of the road, the traffic conditions or the weather ahead – all of which might impact on how quickly we might reach the destination indicated by the milestone marker. Thus, we need to be cautious about using delays in the acquisition of motor milestones as the only indicator of motor 'problems' without considering additional information.

These additional perspectives should include observations about the quality of the motor performance. Thus, for example, a child of 12 months who is not pulling to stand but who crawls actively on all fours with good reciprocal movements of their limbs is demonstrating solid integration of motor control and will certainly walk without difficulty, even if at that particular age they are 'failing' to reach a classic motor milestone of walking at 12 months. Here one is using the knowledge that the presence of well-coordinated hip control is an essential – and in this example well-developed – component of bipedal mobility.

On the other hand, one might see a 12-month-old who pulls to stand and perhaps cruises along the furniture in one direction but cannot crawl and repeatedly flips out of a prone position to avoid crawling. In these circumstances one may be observing a child with a hemisyndrome that is only now becoming evident, affecting the early development of motor skills that require symmetrical motor control. This is a child who may walk 'late' and may never crawl well (or indeed at all) but whose gross motor prognosis is probably quite good.

It is important to recognize that in the early stages of the 'development' and presentation of CP, even experts may be uncertain about whether a young child's motor function difficulties are in fact 'CP'. Under these circumstances, it may be very appropriate for a physician to recognize that this is a story 'in progress', to acknowledge that the young person does indeed have difficulties and to make a referral to an experienced developmental (usually physical) therapist. The goals at this point will include problem-based advice for parents about the 'handling' and 'management' of the young person (see Bower 2008; Dodd et al. 2010). This is also an opportunity to use the next weeks and months to assess what changes happen as the child continues to develop. As suggested earlier, reassessment after an appropriate period of time will allow clinicians to take advantage of the 'test of time' in order to gain the perspectives afforded by the opportunity for further development. This will provide information about the emergence of the young child's individual patterns of motor (and other developmental) function.

Comprehensive clinical and functional assessments

Models for the comprehensive assessment of children with neurological disabilities have been in existence for at least 40 years. As early as the 1970s, the creation of developmental disability teams explicitly recognized that the expertise that is required in the comprehensive assessment of disabled children, and perhaps especially CP, is not derived from any single profession or professional. In consequence, assessment teams have varied in composition, organization, location and working methods.

In the UK, the status of hospital-based child development teams, child development centres and similarly named bodies has largely been overtaken by centring services in the community and by encouraging active parental involvement in the assessment process. This has occurred in part as a consequence of policies aimed at strengthening community services. This development has limited the role of tertiary hospital-based paediatric neurology services so that these now supplement and advise community paediatric services.

Despite the implication that there will be community provision for the assessment of children with CP and other disabilities, there are no models of practice that have an accepted or established validity. It follows that teams' membership varies in terms of the types of professional involved and also their degree of knowledge and experience.

For example, in the UK and especially with respect to physiotherapy, occupational therapy, and speech and language therapy professionals, no formal paediatric or disability qualifications are mandatory before practitioners can work in this field. While the vast majority of therapists who work with disabled children have obtained experience in junior posts, only some will have obtained specific and focused qualifications (for example, in paediatric dysphagia).

In Canada, many service programmes are publicly funded and community based, such that children with CP rarely come to hospital except for acute illnesses or surgery. As in the UK, professionals who work with disabled children are usually pursuing an active career choice. In fact, in larger urban areas professional positions in childhood disability programmes are often hard to find because they are so popular.

Members of the multiprofessional team who are concerned with the assessment of CP and other disabilities vary according to profession and expertise. Teams may include individuals with experience in preschool teaching, paediatric nursing, health visiting, play therapy and clinical psychology. Some teams include expertise in assessment of hearing and of vision. Where no paediatric expertise is available, it can be a major challenge to have children's hearing and vision evaluated appropriately.

The assessment for schooling should be part of the comprehensive assessment of a child with CP. Here the role of the educational psychologist is particularly important. We consider that careful assessment of children's cognitive and social abilities is mandatory. We would also make the point that there are purpose-designed clinical tools and assessments that should be used, both for consistency and communication and because these tools address issues specific to CP (e.g. the Quality FM [Wright, 2011, personal communication]). Space does not permit a comprehensive list of CP-specific assessment tools, but some are discussed in Chapter 12.

Optimally there should also always be a low threshold for obtaining more specialist advice. Examples include advice that is available from paediatric neurology, from specialist feeding, from spasticity management and from paediatric orthopaedic surgical services. In the UK there is also some limited provision of specialist therapy advice. This list is not meant to be exhaustive and could include advice from specialist mental health services and specialist educational services.

We would also emphasize that the purpose of the assessment is first to formulate a comprehensive but comprehensible description of the issues, and second to provide short- and medium-term planning with the family. Within this context, no single profession or professional owns or necessarily should always lead this process. It is often the case that it is helpful to have a key worker (*CanChild* 2005), whether specifically designated or not, and preferably selected by the parents. This professional can act as a coordinator of services and, if need be, also as an advocate for the family.

Implications for practice: wrapping up the consultation assessment

After recognizing that a child is presenting with clinical features consistent with a diagnostic label of CP, what is done and said next, and what is best fed back to a family, depends on the questions that have initially been posed to the clinician. Where clinicians work in teams, it is particularly important to have as consistent a 'house style' as possible. Few things have more potential for creating confusion for families than for a paediatrician to use the phrase 'brain damage', a physiotherapist to use the phrase 'CP' and an orthopaedic surgeon to use the description 'quadriplegia' in consultations about the same child. These variations in terminology – all of which are accurate terms but substantially different words – can create an impression that a child has multiple 'diseases' when this is of course not the case. The use of these multiple labels can also convey the impression that members of the team do not communicate effectively.

Hence, the messages that need to be got across include confirmation that there are neurological impairments; that these include abnormalities of movement and motor function; that the generic phrase CP is commonly used to explain what this entails, individualized for their child; that time is available for further discussion; and that a programme for assistance to be undertaken in partnership with the family will be initiated. Communication at this stage – both in person and in writing – should principally be with the family. It should be as detailed and as free of jargon as possible. The report should, with consent, be distributed to relevant health and other professionals.

References

Al-Qabandi M, Gorter JW, Rosenbaum P (2011) Early autism detection: are we ready for routine screening? *Pediatrics* 128: e211.

Bower E (2008) *Handling the Young Child with Cerebral Palsy at Home*. Oxford: Butterworth-Heinemann.

CanChild, Drennan A, Wagner T, Rosenbaum P (2005) The 'key worker' model of service delivery. Available at: http://www.canchild.ca/en/canchildresources/keyworker.asp.

Cans C (2000) Surveillance of cerebral palsy in Europe: a collaboration of cerebral palsy surveys and registers. *Dev Med Child Neurol* 42: 816–24.

Cioni G, Mercuri E (2008) *Neurological Assessment in the First Two Years of Life*. Clinics in Developmental Medicine No. 176. London: Mac Keith Press.

Day SM, Brooks J, Shumway S, Strauss D, Rosenbloom L (2012) Growth charts for children with cerebral palsy: weight and stature percentiles by age, gender, and level of disability. In: Preedy VR, editor, *Handbook of Growth and Growth Monitoring in Health and Disease*, Part 10. New York: Springer, pp. 1675–1709.

Dodd K, Imms C, Taylor NF (2010) *Physiotherapy and Occupational Therapy for People with Cerebral Palsy: A Problem-Based Approach to Assessment and Management*. London: Mac Keith Press.

Einspieler C, Prechtl HRF, Bos A, Ferrari F, Cioni G (2005) *Prechtl's Method on the Qualitative Assessment of General Movements in Preterm, Term and Young Infants.* Clinics in Developmental Medicine No. 167. London: Mac Keith Press.

Eliasson A, Krumlinde-Sundholm L, Rösblad E et al. (2006) The Manual Ability Classification System (MACS) for children with cerebral palsy: scale development and evidence of validity and reliability. *Dev Med Child Neurol* 48: 549–59.

Gage JR, Schwartz MH, Koop SE, Novacheck TF (2009) *The Identification and Treatment of Gait Problems in Cerebral Palsy,* 2nd edn. Clinics in Developmental Medicine 180–181. London: Mac Keith Press.

King MD, Stephenson JBP (2009) *A Handbook of Neurological Investigations in Children.* London: Mac Keith Press.

Levene MI, Chervenak FA (2009) *Fetal and Neonatal Neurology and Neurosurgery,* 4th edn. Edinburgh: Churchill Livingstone.

McIntosh N, Helms P, Smyth R, Logan S, editors (2008) *Forfar and Arneil's Textbook of Pediatrics.* Edinburgh: Elsevier.

Morris C, Dias L (2007) *Paediatric Orthotics.* Clinics in Developmental Medicine No. 175. London: Mac Keith Press.

Palisano RJ, Rosenbaum P, Bartlett D, Livingston MH (2008) Content validity of the expanded and revised Gross Motor Function Classification System. *Dev Med Child Neurol* 50: 744–50.

Rennie JM, Hagmann CF, Robertson NJ (2008) *Neonatal Cerebral Investigation,* 2nd edn. Cambridge: Cambridge University Press.

Rosenbaum PL (2006a) Classification of abnormal neurological outcome. *Early Hum Dev* 82: 167–71.

Rosenbaum PL (2006b) Variation and 'abnormality': recognizing the differences. Invited editorial. *J Pediatr* 149: 593–4.

Rosenbaum PL, Missiuna C, Echeverria D, Knox SS (2009) Proposed motor development assessment protocol for epidemiological studies in children. *J Epidemiol Community Health* 63: i27–i36.

Russman BS, Ashwal S (2004) Evaluation of the child with cerebral palsy. *Semin Pediatr Neurol* 11: 47–57.

Sanger TD, Delgado MR, Gaebler-Spira, D, Hallett M, Mink JW; Task Force on Childhood Motor Disorders (2003) Classification and definition of disorders causing hypertonia in childhood. *Pediatrics* 111: e89–e97.

Sanger TD, Chen D, Fehlings DL et al. (2010) Definition and classification of hyperhinetic movements in childhood. *Mov Disord* 25: 1538–49.

Chapter 10

Principles of interventions

Overview

Recognizing that there is an underlying brain abnormality is the catalyst for both parents and professionals to examine the range of possible interventions that may be of benefit to a child with cerebral palsy (CP). In this chapter we examine first the principles that underlie the interventions that are considered, rightly or wrongly, to promote function and adjustment of children with CP and, second, those that may promote parental adaptation. In doing so we examine concepts of brain plasticity, the possibility of whether nervous tissue can recover after being injured and measures that may prevent further brain injury. Third, we describe the principles of the habilitative approaches that are used to improve or maintain function or to prevent deterioration, and the contexts in which these may be applied. Against these backgrounds, we discuss how promotion of adaptation on the part of children, their families and treating professionals may be achieved, and the relevance of quality of life issues. Finally we attempt to put all of these ideas together within the overall context of the principles of service delivery.

Brain injury and neuronal plasticity

Neuronal plasticity refers to the capacity of the nervous system to be shaped or moulded by experiences. The subject is well discussed by Rimrodt and Johnston (2009). Neuronal plasticity can be defined as 'the state of still having several options for specialization left within the developmental process'. While the bulk of plasticity in the typically developing individual is seen in young infants, there is also evidence that it extends to a degree into adult life.

A variety of cellular and physiological mechanisms contribute to plasticity in the developing brain, and four types of clinical plasticity are described. These are *adaptive* plasticity used in acquiring new skills; *impaired* plasticity such as is seen in intellectual disability; *excessive* plasticity, for example the development of abnormal neuronal circuits in hippocampal sclerosis and temporal lobe epilepsy; and plasticity that creates a *vulnerability to injury*. An example of this last one is the effect of glutamate release after perinatal hypoxic–ischaemia, leading ultimately to excitotoxic cell death.

The implication of work on neuronal plasticity is that it can form a basis for the use of neuroprotective regimens in infants and children who are thought to have been subject to recent brain injury. These include the use of hypothermia (Shankaran et al. 2005) in asphyxiated term-born infants together with more experimental approaches including the use of stem cell replacement therapy. What needs to be emphasized, however, is that there is a very limited time window for the institution of any neuroprotective regimen.

A further issue with respect to brain plasticity is the tension between the ability of the damaged brain to develop or re-establish functions that have been lost, for example regaining language after hemispherectomy of the dominant hemisphere, and the likelihood that there will be evolving evidence of progressively more overt impairments with age. This is seen, for example, when there has been frontal lobe damage in a young person but where executive functioning impairments that derive from this damage can be tested only in adolescence and adult life.

Translation of these concepts into clinical practice is difficult because it is not possible to generalize to individual children from what has been learned from studies involving groups, populations or animals. This is discussed further below when considering the principles that are used in advising our approach to discussing available interventions.

Principles of service delivery

Throughout this book we have tried to emphasize several ideas that we see to be fundamental to our work with children with CP and their families. Perhaps first among these is the importance of taking a strengths-based approach to the child and family – seeing capability rather than disability (*CanChild* 2003a). It is essential to ask the family about what they consider to be the things in their life that are 'working', and to use those assets in our discussions and recommendations to them. We have in mind issues like a child's cheerful personality (part of who that person is); the child's ability to do things, even if they do them 'differently' (as opposed to the all too frequent compiling of a catalogue of what the child cannot do); the availability of family resources like grandparents and other extended family who can provide time, financial help and emotional support; and friends who accept the child and family despite the child's disability. It is important not to take these and many other strengths for granted, but to both ask about and celebrate them as part of what the family brings with them on their journey into the new world of childhood disability.

We have described in some detail why we believe it is important to be attentive to the views and needs of parents and families. In Chapter 8 we discuss, among several related themes, communication with families. It will therefore be apparent that we consider that a basic principle of all our clinical activities is the need to work in partnership with parents and families. Family-centred services (also outlined in Chapter 8) provide a framework within which this can be done.

We have also discussed (in Chapter 7) the concepts embedded within the World Health Organization (WHO)'s International Classification of Functioning, Disability and Health (ICF) framework (World Health Organization 2001). In particular, we believe that it is essential to take a practical and 'functional' approach to 'treatment' and management (Rosenbaum and Gorter 2011), and not to assume that interventions directed at impairments will necessarily lead to changes in function. Indeed, work by Wright and her colleagues (Wright et al. 2007) has shown that such an assumption does not hold up to careful scrutiny.

Another principle of modern service delivery is the importance, wherever possible, of considering how our recommendations – and our actual services – take account of the environments (both local and community based) that are important to children and families. This idea not only is responsive to notions of family-centredness, but also recognizes the role that 'environments' play in the expression of people's capacity to participate in daily life. With respect to the larger community environment, we know that the participation of children with CP is influenced by where they live (Hammal et al. 2004; Fauconnier et al. 2009) as well as by a family's socioeconomic status (Law et al. 2006).

As but one interesting example, environmental setting has been shown to exert a powerful effect on the methods of usual mobility of children with CP (Palisano et al. 2003; Tieman et al. 2004a,b). In addition, mobility in daily life is influenced by age as well as by environmental factors (Palisano et al. 2010). We also know that the expression of people's 'capacity' (what we can do at our best) is significantly impacted by factors external to the person, such that environmental supports and barriers influence our actual day-to-day 'performance'. Morris (2009) refers to people's 'capability' as being, in effect, a product of person–environment interaction.

We need to remember that when we do a formal assessment of a child's performance, we are trying to observe their best capacity under the best environmental circumstances. For example, in the clinic we try to look at a child's mobility in a physical setting designed to facilitate mobility, with parental encouragement, counting on the child's desire to please. This is important because it provides an indication of what we assume to be best abilities, and allows us to have an idea of the functional goals for which we will strive.

However, it is too easy to assume that the capacity that we see in clinic is what children will accomplish in their community settings. Continuing the example of mobility, environment factors such as the nature and quality of walking surfaces, crowding and time limitations (such as needing to move from one classroom to another quickly) may all significantly influence what people actually do, and how well they do it (i.e. their performance in the real world).

For all of these reasons it is important that our services be attentive to community realities. A recent excellent measure of mobility (the Functional Mobility Scale; Graham et al. 2004) explicitly looks at a child's performance in three environments – home, school and the community. Being able to see people in these familiar environments provides perspectives that we know are invaluable. When we can see children in their home environments, we see them where they are probably most comfortable, and where young children in particular spend a lot of time. This exposure also makes it possible to understand the constraints of the environment and to help parents take advantage of the opportunities afforded by that specific environment. It has been shown that assessments done in the home provide information that is as useful as that achieved in a clinic setting (Rosenbaum et al. 1990).

Ideal versus real: are these ideas practical?
The authors are sensitive to the probability that in many circumstances there will be disparities between what service providers would wish to see done and what is possible for a child, a family or a service system. Several factors probably come into play to influence this reality. First, there may be limitations in the amount and quality of resources available in one's community to address and help manage the challenges faced by a child and family. These resource limitations may involve the medical, educational, recreational and social service sectors. There are no easy answers for this situation. One must simply be creative and not be constrained or daunted by what is missing.

A second factor that may contribute to what is and is not available is politics – be they related to medical, therapy, education or other services. There are often discrepancies in services between conditions that are 'popular' and those that get less attention in the media or from the many support systems that are expected to be available. One approach to address this reality is to take a human rights perspective and to argue for equity for all children regardless of disorder or diagnostic label.

There is considerable value in taking a 'non-categorical' approach to the shared needs of children with neurodisabilities and their families and in recognizing the potential for strength in numbers that is possible when families pool their energies. In this way of thinking, the common developmental, educational and social elements across conditions are recognized and emphasized. This tactic is distinct from the important individualized biomedical focus on the identification of a precise 'diagnosis' in each case, whereby specific medical, genetic and prognostic factors should be identified and acted on.

Third, the training and expertise of professionals varies from place to place and over time. This means, among other things, that the amount and quality of parental support and education may be very varied across a community and appear to be 'unfair'. Both parents and professionals need to be aware of what the effective services look like and lobby appropriately (and hopefully in concert) to improve the situation.

Finally, in some places even the basic availability of services depends on the expectation that professionals will be able to provide evidence of 'success' of services like those that are needed but are insufficiently available. This begs the question about what 'outcomes' the resource manager or policy-maker wants, and why. As is argued in many places in this book, these are challenging issues, and often the evidence to support the value of services is simply not available because the right studies have not yet been done. Furthermore, a very reasonable goal for many people might be maintenance of health or functional status, where a lack of change over time represents success. This is a particularly complex idea for many people, and speaks to the important need for good longitudinal studies of the 'natural history' of the health and functional status of people with CP with which to argue how maintenance of a person's status is important.

Regarding intervention goals, we have argued throughout this book and elsewhere (Rosenbaum 2009) that the broad focus of all our work with disabled children should be on promoting children's development. To the extent that we have interventions for people with CP that are known to be effective – be they physical (e.g. therapies), educational, biomedical (e.g. drugs and surgery) or technical (e.g. braces, computers, walking aids) – we certainly should use them if they will enhance function. An important example of a technical intervention (powered mobility) that led to powerful impacts on children's functioning is provided by the work of Butler (1986).

There should always be a functional goal in mind, and wherever possible an assessment of whether our interventions are 'working' (against predefined goals) should be undertaken. We must also be prepared to change the goals as the previous targets are either achieved or reconsidered over time. In other words, our eye should always be on the 'so what' question regarding whether any intervention can be shown to have an effect on actual performance (or at least an excellent likelihood of doing so). This perspective differs quite a lot from traditional beliefs that therapies should be directed at underlying 'impairments' in the hope that addressing and improving the impairment will lead to functional improvement. This may indeed be true, but the strength of the argument should be based on evidence rather than belief alone.

In our conversations with parents, we encourage them to take a long-term view of their child's journey through childhood. We remind them that the adult world imposes on all children the expectation (at least in school) that they try to perform in a very wide range of areas. Adults expect children to learn and hopefully demonstrate skills in many activities – be they social, physical, intellectual, artistic – that are much more demanding than what most adults ever expect of themselves, or ever perform, on a day-to-day basis. We want to help parents to recognize that if they can help their children weather the childhood years with these many and varied demands (demands which also often challenge many children without disabilities), the children will have the opportunity to define themselves effectively as competent people rather than as 'damaged goods'.

The point of the argument is that we should encourage parents to strive to help their children, in the course of their developing years, to develop competencies, interests and a sense of self-confidence despite their 'disabilities', because after the childhood years they will have many more opportunities to find their niche in life.

A related aspect of goal setting concerns which goals should be articulated and pursued. Traditionally, professionals were the acknowledged experts, and it was we who set the intervention agenda. This clearly makes sense in so far as we bring to the discussion our experience and perspectives on CP. We are in a position to propose interventions that are known or believed to be effective, and to tailor our advice to the specific child and family issues. However, as discussed elsewhere, traditional models of intervention have addressed 'impairments' in body function and structure, with the assumption that these needed to be remediated ('normalized'), and that changes in impairments would translate to improvements in function.

As discussed in more detail in Chapter 8, in an era that values a family-centred approach, and with the assumption that we should be mindful of parents' values and goals, we believe that goal setting should be a shared activity between parents and professionals. This approach is respectful of parents: it promotes partnership, it acknowledges parents as the world's expert on their child and it is much more likely to lead to the articulation of practical functional goals that will be addressed by parents' adherence to recommended treatment. An excellent randomized clinical trial by Ketelaar and colleagues (2001) demonstrated clearly that when therapists provided services to address parent- or child-identified goals, the outcomes were better than those achieved when children were treated to achieve therapist-defined goals – and with less intervention.

Treating the whole child: general issues

It is axiomatic that a fundamental principle of intervention in children (and adults) with CP is that there should be a focus on general health issues as there is with any other child. Depending on the nature and extent of the neurological impairments, affected individuals can demonstrate the whole range of health problems that may be seen in the general population, together with some specific issues that are more likely to occur because of, and in association with, the individual having CP.

The most important of these special issues relates to growth and nutrition (Day et al. 2007). Both as a direct consequence of brain damage and also mediated by dietary, feeding, swallowing and other difficulties, children with CP commonly demonstrate varying degrees of nutritional failure. This is discussed further in Chapter 11.

One aspect of treatment that requires consideration is that, against the background of CP arising as a consequence of a non-progressive brain damage, it is nevertheless important to consider the possibility of further brain damage occurring. This comes to mind when there is regression of previous abilities (even if they have already been impaired). In clinical practice, this may be seen after very severe intercurrent illnesses, especially if a period of ventilator support for respiratory failure has been needed. Under that circumstance there is a risk that cerebral perfusion failure may add to pre-existing brain damage. Refractory seizures or status epilepticus also carry a small risk of exacerbating the degree of neurological impairment, as do episodes of raised intracranial pressure in children whose CP is seen in association with them also having shunt-dependent hydrocephalus.

Other health and developmental issues that require addressing include the diagnosis and management of concurrent epilepsy in children with CP, the recognition and management of visual and hearing impairments, the evaluation of any cognitive or communication impairments and of their significance to the child's overall functioning, and the evaluation of the whole range of possible behavioural and somatic symptom-atology. Specific focus is often required on the nature and source of perceived pain in children with impaired communication, and on sleep behaviours, especially when there are reported sleep disturbances.

Disagreements between parents and service providers

Given differences in perspectives between parents and professionals, and indeed across professionals, disagreements are likely to arise about goals and the best means to achieve them. Regarding disagreements between parents and professionals, it is already apparent that we consider that it is important to respect parents' goals to the greatest extent possible. This includes engaging with parents in goal setting, as outlined in Chapter 12.

There can be a number of other bases for parents to disagree with professionals, and vice versa. The reasons may be practical – for example, parents perceiving that their child is not getting enough therapy, or for professionals believing that parents are not following through well enough on therapy recommendations. Parents may be frus-trated if they fail to see the effects of the treatments they are doing. Stretching muscles is an excellent example of something that is often recommended, but can be taxing for parents, uncomfortable for children and of uncertain (or at least unobserved) benefit. Needless to say, a family-centred approach to the negotiation of these tricky issues is strongly recommended (*CanChild* 2003b).

Some people believe that in the context of family-centred service, professionals must accede to parents' wishes on all issues. This is clearly a distortion of the notion of respectful partnerships with parents. While respecting parents' ideas and requests, professionals have a responsibility to counsel families about the possible implications of what we consider to be inappropriate goals or treatments. We are also under no obligation to pursue treatments we know to be useless or harmful. When disagreements arise, the issues and ideas should be discussed openly and people should be allowed to disagree (Rosenbaum 1997; Rosenbaum and Stewart 2002). It is important to keep the door open, especially when parents are pursuing complementary and alternative therapies that we believe will produce disappointing outcomes. It is important for parents to know that they can return to our orbit at any time.

When professionals disagree, it is important that we discuss the issues openly and avoid power struggles, especially those based on sex or profession (we mention these in particular because they are often at the root of disagreements). We should have recourse to the literature and the 'evidence', avoiding anecdotes in favour of more reasoned argument. Professional disagreements should, wherever possible, be played out behind the scenes so that parents are not caught in the middle and forced to take sides or divide their loyalties. At the same time, it is important for parents to know that in fields like childhood neurodisability, where sound evidence is often lacking, honest differences of opinion can be constructive opportunities for everyone concerned to explore the issues and seek the best currently available answer. This highlights the need for clear communication between all professionals and use of common language.

Disability as 'deprivation'

One way to conceptualize the idea of childhood disabilities is to recognize the potential for children's functional limitations to lead them to experience 'deprivation'. What we mean here is not parental neglect, although of course that should always be considered in children who are failing to make as much progress as we expect. Rather, we refer to the ways in which the constraints on a child's functional capacity may limit their opportunities for the self-generated activity and exploration that are such an essential aspect of children's 'incidental' learning. We also recognize that many parents have competing demands on their time and resources and might not be able to do as much for their children as they would wish. This should not, in our opinion, be construed as 'neglect'.

In considering the idea of 'deprivation' in disability, one need simply think about a typical 2-year-old's mobility to recognize how easily mobility restrictions in a child with CP can constrain their experience and hence their development. Among the reasons adults refer to children of this age as 'terrible' is the children's perpetual busyness. They constantly use their emerging gross and fine motor capacity, along with their emerging language and other skills, to explore their world – to run and jump and climb and touch and experiment – all in the service of development.

Imagine, then, how a child experiencing a mobility restriction (or any other functional limitation) may be 'deprived' by their inability to engage in these relentless pursuits of exploration. Unless we incorporate this developmental perspective into our thinking and plan interventions that accommodate the child's restrictions, we are missing opportunities to promote active learning. This idea illustrates how concerns about treating 'disability' need to intersect with our interest in child development.

The work of Butler (1986) cited earlier is a superb illustration of the way that a technical intervention (powered mobility), targeting activity rather than impairments, literally and figuratively empowered 2- and 3-year-old children with severe mobility restrictions. There were huge changes in play, social function, communication and exploration ('participation' in the WHO's ICF terminology) made by these children within weeks of receiving a power wheelchair. These improvements encourage the opportunity to intervene at a developmental level, to overcome experiential limitations and to prevent at least some of the secondary deprivation associated with neurodisabilities (Rosenbaum 2008).

This component of an approach to intervention needs to be discussed with parents. They may need help to understand that 'parenting is a dance led by the children'. What we mean by this is that a very large element of parenting is reactive – parents are constantly trying to keep up with and adapt to the developmental and behavioural manifestations of their typical children's ever-changing capacity. If we accept that, as a result of their functional limitations, many disabled children may not be able to 'dance' well, we identify a major challenge in parenting disabled children. When, as we have often done, we 'prescribe mischief' and explain these developmental ideas to parents, they catch the spirit of the idea and can more easily contrive to allow and encourage their children's natural curiosity to emerge, in whatever ways might be appropriate, before learned helplessness and secondary disabilities take root.

These ideas speak to the importance of a strengths-based approach to all our work with parents of disabled children. It is too easy to catalogue the child's problems and limitations and to fail to ask parents what they are happy about regarding their child's status and function. We need to encourage parents to notice, value and focus on their child's and family's strengths. We need to build our whole intervention philosophy and strategy around such an approach.

In some approaches to intervention in CP there have at times been admonitions that children not be 'allowed' or encouraged to do things 'wrongly' or 'abnormally'. It is quite probable that restrictions like these contributed to the differences in outcomes observed in one of the early clinical trial interventions in CP (Palmer et al. 1988). In that study, children in an infant development programme, apparently given free rein to explore and be active, functioned better in motor skills at 6 and 12 months than did children receiving neurodevelopmental therapy.

As well intentioned as these admonitions may have been, we believe that they are too restrictive and need to be either well evaluated as being valid or abandoned in favour of a freer approach to encouraging child function. We discuss (in Chapter 13) the functional value of W-sitting for some children as an illustration of 'allowing' children to find their own best ways to achieve function. This also highlights the importance of understanding that a child does things in many ways, for example using a variety of ways of sitting. W-sitting is all right if we are providing other activities to balance out the less ideal elements of this activity.

Here as elsewhere there may be tension between traditional attention to the biomedical impairments and the current emphasis on function and achievement. Such tensions are a waste of energy and can be counterproductive. We value any impairment-based interventions that are known to 'work'. We also value interventions and activities that promote children's development. We see these approaches as potentially complementary – as long as the biomedical interventions do not lead to restrictions on what the developing child wants, and is able, to do. And of course an approach that encourages free-range function does not preclude the use of relevant biomedical and technical interventions that support the achievement of the child's goals.

An example where tension could arise might be the recommendation that a child should be wearing night splints, or a spinal jacket to correct or perhaps to prevent a skeletal malalignment. As service providers we need to be able to offer a clear rationale and hopefully sound evidence of the probable benefits of what may be seen by parents as a cumbersome, uncomfortable and perhaps expensive intervention. There should also be a measurable outcome that is agreed to by parents and professionals and a time frame within which these outcomes will be measured. There can also be a previous agreement about what the course of action should be, depending on the outcome observed.

Don't judge the book by the cover
It will already be clear that we believe that it is essential to assess children carefully, noting both their capacities and the functional difficulties they are experiencing. There are a couple of reasons why this is important. First, given that children are assessed and managed because of functional problems, it is too easy for professionals to focus on deficits to the exclusion of the rest of the child's status. This easily leads us to characterize the child in terms of their impairments and limitations, and in turn channels discussions with parents towards this side of the child's life.

Second, the identification of capacities is important as a way of determining how best to encourage a child's development by capitalizing on those strengths. As discussed earlier in this chapter, it is essential that parents are encouraged to view their children as whole people – with strengths and capacities as well as problems. When we look for and articulate this side of a child's being, we reinforce the importance of this idea.

There is a widely acknowledged covariance of neurodevelopmental challenges additional to motor difficulties in people with CP. In fact, these ideas influenced the 2007 revision of the definition of CP and are captured in the second sentence (Rosenbaum et al. 2007). However, these epidemiological correlations should not automatically be generalized to a specific child. A difficulty in one area of development should not be assumed to be a marker for problems in other areas. Each child should be assessed systematically and their individual constellation of functional abilities and needs should be noted carefully.

There may be a tendency for well-meaning professionals to make unrealistic estimates of the capabilities (or, indeed, the limitations) of disabled children with CP. We strongly recommend that people describe what they observe in the various dimensions of functioning – mobility, communication, social function, and cognitive and academic performance – so that others with the appropriate expertise can use these valuable observations as a basis for making specific interpretations and judgements. Parents and professionals such as teachers and other community-based people have the special opportunity to see children outside of the clinic setting and can offer very useful information simply by reporting carefully what they observe rather than interpreting the 'facts' too fully.

In addition, it will be apparent that as children grow and develop, this assessment needs to be current. Reliance on parental report – and encouraging parents to brag about their child – can enable us to be aware of the emerging abilities and personal traits that become such an essential part of each child's unique picture.

Promoting adaptation

We have suggested that in counselling parents, it is important to take a long view of their child's and family's journey through the developing years. Some parents (and indeed some professionals) need to be reminded that there are no miracle cures for the impairments that underlie the functional challenges experienced by people with CP. While there may be no hope for a cure, there is much that can be done to enhance child and family development and well-being.

Children are in a constant state of 'becoming'. It is essential to help parents to promote their children's competence, capability, sense of self and independence to the greatest extent possible. Much is being written about 'quality of life', and these issues are discussed in more detail in Chapter 14. At this point we are simply highlighting that what we refer to as the 'existential' aspect of quality of life is, in our opinion, distinctly different from functional status or 'health-related quality of life'. Thus, people may feel very comfortable within their own skin 'despite' functional limitations that, to an outsider, might be assumed to constrain one's 'quality' of life. It is important to distinguish self-assessment from the judgements and values of others.

We believe that in part this starts with the tone we set in our early counselling with families and continues over time through the open and honest relationships we establish with them (as described in Chapter 8). Our optimism should reflect the expectation that we can help parents to parent effectively even when their child has a disability.

Finally, it will be apparent that the approach to intervention advocated in this chapter emphasizes the need to reach a balance on a number of themes. We recommend a focus on functional achievement rather than solely on trying to fix impairments. We seek to promote children's development without expecting 'normal' performance, and we certainly do not wish to see children held back from doing things because their performance is less than perfect. We value and recommend a partnership with parents so that our therapeutic goals reflect their ideas as well as our advice. This is the climate we should seek to establish, within which the specific intervention strategies are provided.

References

Butler C (1986) Effects of powered mobility on self-initiated behaviours of very young children with locomotor disability. *Dev Med Child Neurol* 28: 325–32.

CanChild (2003a) Fact Sheet #6. Available at: http://www.canchild.ca/en/childrenfamilies/resources/FCSSheet6.pdf.

CanChild (2003b) Fact Sheet #11. Available at: http://www.canchild.ca/en/childrenfamilies/resources/FCSSheet11.pdf.

Day SM, Strauss DJ, Vachon PJ, Rosenbloom, L, Shavelle RM, Wu YW (2007) Growth patterns in a population of children and adolescents with cerebral palsy. *Dev Med Child Neurol* 49: 167–71.

Fauconnier J, Dickinson HO, Beckung E et al. (2009) Participation in life situations of 8–12 year old children with cerebral palsy: cross sectional European study. *BMJ* 338: b1458.

Graham HK, Harvey A, Rodda J, Nattrass GR, Pirpiris M (2004) The Functional Mobility Scale (FMS). *J Pediatr Orthop* 24: 514–20.

Hammal D, Jarvis SN, Colver AF (2004) Participation of children with cerebral palsy is influenced by where they live [see comment]. *Dev Med Child Neurol* 46: 292–8.

Ketelaar M, Vermeer A, Hart H, van Petegem-van Beek E, Helders PJ (2001) Effects of a functional therapy program on motor abilities of children with cerebral palsy. *Phys Ther* 81: 1534–45

Law M, King G, King S, Kertoy M et al. (2006) Patterns of participation in recreational and leisure activities among children with complex physical disabilities. *Dev Med Child Neurol* 48: 337–42.

Morris C (2009) Measuring participation in childhood disability: how does the capability approach improve our understanding? *Dev Med Child Neurol* 51: 92–4.

Palisano RJ, Hanna SE, Rosenbaum PL, Tieman B (2010) Probability of walking, wheeled mobility, and assisted mobility in children and adolescents with cerebral palsy. *Dev Med Child Neurol* 52: 66–71.

Palisano RJ, Tieman BL, Walter SD et al. (2003) Effect of environmental setting on mobility methods of children with cerebral palsy. *Dev Med Child Neurol* 45: 113–20.

Palmer FB, Shapiro BK, Wachtel RC et al. (1988) The effects of physical therapy on cerebral palsy. A controlled trial in infants with spastic diplegia. *N Engl J Med* 318: 803–8.

Rimrodt S, Johnston MV (2009) Neuronal plasticity and developmental disability. In: *Neurodevelopmental Disabilities: Clinical and Scientific Foundations*, Shevell M (ed.) London: Mac Keith Press.

Rosenbaum PL (1997) 'Alternative' treatments for children with disabilities: thoughts from the trenches. *Paediatr Child Health* 2: 122–4.

Rosenbaum P (2008) Effects of powered mobility on self-initiated behaviours of very young children with locomotor disability. *Dev Med Child Neurol* 50: 644.

Rosenbaum P (2009) Putting child development back into developmental disabilities. *Dev Med Child Neurol* 51: 251.

Rosenbaum PL, Gorter JW (2011) The 'F-words' in childhood disability: I swear this is how we should think! child: care, health and development. doi:10.1111/j.1365-2214.2011.01338.x.

Rosenbaum P, Stewart D (2002) Alternative and complementary therapies for children and youth with disabilities. *Infants Young Child* 15: 51–9.

Rosenbaum P, King S, Toal C (1990) Home or Cerebral Palsy Centre: where should the initial therapy assessments of children with disabilities be done? *Dev Med Child Neurol* 32: 888–94.

Rosenbaum P, Paneth N, Leviton A, Goldstein M, Bax M (2007) Definition and classification document. In: *The Definition and Classification of Cerebral Palsy* Baxter P (ed.) *Dev Med Child Neurol* 49 (Suppl. 2): 8–14.

Shankaran S, Laptook AR, Ehrenkranz RA et al. (2005) National Institute of Child Health and Human Development Neonatal Research Network. Whole-body hypothermia for neonates with hypoxic-ischemic encephalopathy. *N Engl J Med* 353: 1574–84.

Sullivan PB, Lambert B, Rose M, Ford-Adams M, Johnson A, Griffith P (2000) Prevalence and severity of feeding and nutritional problems in children with neurological impairment: Oxford Feeding Study. *Dev Med Child Neurol* 42: 10–80.

Tieman B, Palisano RJ, Gracely EJ, Rosenbaum PL (2004a) Gross motor capability and performance of mobility in children with cerebral palsy: a comparison across home, school, and outdoors/community settings. *Phys Ther* 84: 419–29.

Tieman BL, Palisano RJ, Gracely EJ, Rosenbaum P, Chairello LA, O'Neil ME (2004b) Changes in mobility of children with cerebral palsy over time and across environmental setting. *Phys Occup Ther Pediatr* 24: 109–28.

World Health Organization (2011) *International Classification of Functioning, Disability and Health.* Geneva: World Health Organization.

Wright FV, Rosenbaum PL, Fehlings D (2007) How do changes in impairment, activity, and participation relate to each other? Study of children with cerebral palsy (CP) who have received lower extremity botulinum toxin type-A (Bt-A) injections. *Dev Med Child Neurol* 50: 283–9.

Chapter 11

Interventions: orthodox and heterodox. A perspective on issues in 'treatment'

with Margaret Mayston

Overview

Two companion chapters discuss 'therapies' and other interventions. This is the first, which provides a broad overview of issues, including health concerns that need to be considered when working with a child and family to plan and implement services. The second (Chapter 12) is focused more specifically on the roles and activities of 'therapists' and the approaches they use to support the development of children with cerebral palsy (CP) and their families.

In the current chapter we first argue that it is important to address general and specific health issues for both children and adults who have CP. Some health problems are usually overt, such as epilepsy, respiratory compromise and impaired nutritional status. Others may be more covert, such as decreased bone density, degenerative joint changes and the risk of myelopathy. Over and above these issues, we recognize that a variety of medical and surgical interventions are commonly used in CP, for example in the management of spasticity, dystonia and involuntary movements, drooling and gastro-oesophageal reflux. Where relevant, these are considered briefly in both this chapter and Chapter 12.

Second, addressing therapies, education and interventions more widely, we make the point that it is very important to learn from our past thinking and experience. We need to beware of orthodoxies that do not allow or encourage intellectual challenge or the testing of ideas with sound clinical science. We must be especially wary of schools of thought that are litigious or that bully anyone who asks questions or challenges beliefs.

Where to begin: the need for skilled human resources

We believe that people who work with children with CP should have appropriate training, experience and expertise in 'applied child development'. Children with 'developmental' disabilities such as CP may phenotypically resemble adults with conditions such as strokes or spinal cord injuries. There are, however, fundamentally important differences between early-onset childhood disabilities that affect the trajectory of a child's (and family's) development and conditions that start in the adult years. Adult-onset disabilities may be equally functionally challenging, but they happen to a person who has previously had adequate capacity, that is a particular level of daily function that provides a guide to what their functional 'rehabilitation' aims to achieve in returning them to their pre-illness status. This reality speaks to the essential difference between the 'rehabilitation' of someone with an adult-onset disability and our 'developmental' work with children with CP and other neurodisabilities (Rosenbaum 2009).

To elaborate briefly on these ideas: in an adult, the broad goals of intervention are based on an effort to *restore* functional abilities. The directions of therapy are guided to a considerable extent by the person's *previous* capacity and their self-identified therapy goals in order to return as closely as possible to the previous state of being and functioning. In contrast, when working with children we strive to promote, support and enhance 'development' – the process of becoming. We consider that an understanding of child and family development is fundamentally important for people who work with children and families. Having an awareness of the natural history and evolution of developmental differences allows people with these perspectives to refrain from 'treating' in situations that have a good prospect of evolving and resolving naturally. (For example, toe walking in an otherwise typically developing child can be ignored and not 'treated'.) In the absence of this experience it is too easy for well-meaning people to intervene in areas where such action may not be warranted, and be distracted by actions that are not needed.

In thinking about interventions for children with CP, one of the many challenges for therapists and parents alike is the need to tailor treatments to individuals in a very careful manner. This is undoubtedly true in other areas of medicine, such as choosing the 'right' anticonvulsant for someone with epilepsy. In this example, the trade-offs are perhaps clearer, involving a choice between stopping seizures and creating new problems with the side effects of the medications.

In the 'management' of CP, however, the goals and end points of 'treatment' are usually less precisely defined than 'seizure control', and are more open to opinion and the 'fashion' of the time. In these circumstances, the choice of therapies can be much more difficult to determine. It is for these reasons that we recommend identifying activity/participation goals based on the World Health Organization (WHO) International Classification of Functioning, Disability and Health (ICF) concepts (see Chapter 7), predetermining relevant end points and trying wherever possible to assess the effectiveness of interventions against these goals within relevant time periods, as described by

Dodd et al. (2010). In other words, it is likely that the specific methods of intervention are generally less important than the skills of the interveners to set appropriate goals with parents (and children where possible) and to recalibrate interventions regularly as functional change and development happen.

This does not mean that the type of method chosen is irrelevant. We are aware that a 'persuasive' intervener who represents even a doubtful/questionable type of intervention can offer what seem to be appropriate goals just by the way that they present them. This highlights the need for parents (and children) to be sure that the goals suggested will directly impact on the child's ability to participate in daily life, and that the steps taken to achieve these goals are compatible with routine family life. We explain more about what we consider to be appropriate goals in the section on 'Resources for intervention' later in this chapter.

Health issues

There are a number of general and specific health issues that are relevant to both children and adults who have CP and that are present to a greater extent than is seen in the unimpaired population. Immobility, communication impairment and dependence are significant factors that contribute to this vulnerability.

Health problems may not always be immediately clinically obvious. They include increased vulnerability to a variety of infections, including those of the respiratory system and the urinary tract. Other problems that should be kept in mind by health and other professionals are issues concerning respiratory function, nutritional status and its maintenance, the management of drooling, bone density issues, the treatment of epilepsy, medical interventions used to manage spasticity, dystonia and involuntary movements, degenerative joint changes and the cervical myelopathy that may be seen in athetoid CP.

In addition, as is summarized in Chapter 12, there is a significant and important role for orthopaedic surgery as a component of multiprofessional therapeutic interventions in CP.

We also emphasize that health issues are not the sole prerogative of doctors and that both parents and all professionals need to have an awareness of their significance. This is important in part because of the adverse effect that health problems exert on well-being, alertness, developmental functioning and the response to other intervention strategies.

It is outside the scope of this book to deal comprehensively with all the relevant health issues that may affect those with CP. Rather we have chosen to summarize some specific illustrative aspects in this chapter and, as has been indicated, we comment on orthopaedic and related interventions for tone disorders and developing deformities in Chapter 12.

Respiratory function

The early clinical features of respiratory infections may be subtle and may merely amount to the child being generally unwell, possibly with an increased respiratory rate.

What we would emphasize, therefore, is that there needs to be an appropriately low threshold for awareness on the part of parents of children with CP, and also on the part of professionals, for the early recognition of a child being 'off colour'. Respiratory infections are more likely to occur if aspiration, which may be silent, occurs in association with receiving food or fluid.

The management of respiratory and other infections is beyond this scope of this discussion. However, for children and adults with CP who have established pulmonary compromise, the involvement of other relevant clinicians is important.

Indeed, at the more severe end of the health spectrum, the most common cause of severe illness and the most common immediate cause of death is pneumonia (Strauss et al. 1999).

Feeding, nutrition and growth in cerebral palsy

It is of particular clinical significance that malnutrition and overt failure to thrive are now seen much less commonly than has historically been the case for children and adults with CP.

The background to this is that there is no reason to think that it is 'normal' for severely disabled children to be small, and it must follow that many have a degree of nutritional impairment consequent upon oromotor difficulties. This is well illustrated in the work of Day et al. (2007). These authors have demonstrated that there is a good correlation between weight and height for age and the degree of disability. Thus, groups of children who are more severely affected in terms of their gross motor and other functions are also lighter and shorter throughout childhood and adolescence.

Moreover, and more recently, Brooks et al. (2011) have also described a correlation with risk of death and impaired nutritional status in children with CP.

Against this background, it is important to emphasize that many children with CP have some degree of feeding difficulty, including a need for help with eating and drinking, a requirement for prolonged mealtimes and frequent vomiting (Sullivan et al. 2009). Indeed, 8% of the children in Sullivan et al.'s (2009) group had a gastrostomy in situ. What is perhaps of greater significance is that more than 64% of the children in this study had not previously received a detailed assessment of their eating, drinking and nutritional status.

Virtually all physiological functions are adversely affected by suboptimal nutrition. Prominent effects include muscle weakness, including weakness of respiratory muscles and hence an enhanced predisposition to chest infections. These effects may also be made more likely by a risk of aspiration of food associated with disordered oromotor control (including swallowing), and by the reduced immunological competence that can be a consequence of impaired nutrition. It may also be that improved nutrition promotes a child's general well-being and alertness and provides an appropriate platform for developmental progress to be made.

In addition to the biomedical components of feeding and nutrition, the psychosocial aspects of feeding disabled children merit consideration. The commitment of parents, especially mothers, to oral feeding can be very strong, sometimes even when there is evidence of very prolonged mealtimes, nutritional failure, signs of aspiration and symptomatic gastro-oesophageal reflux. Careful and sympathetic multidisciplinary assessments and reviews may be required over quite long time periods before definitive plans, for example for gastrostomy feeding, are implemented. It is important to remember as well that for the older person with CP, difficulties with eating and drinking can present a significant challenge to social acceptance.

It follows that an integral component of the investigation and management of children with CP is a multidisciplinary assessment of their oromotor, feeding and nutritional status combined with appropriate investigations, for example videofluoroscopy studies when these are indicated.

This area of practice is described in detail in the text *Feeding and Nutrition in Children with Neurodevelopmental Disability* (Sullivan 2009).

Bone health
Osteoporosis evaluation and its prevention are relevant to children with CP. It has been demonstrated that both bone growth and bone density are frequently impaired in children with CP, and this appears to be related both to the severity of their motor disorder and also to their nutritional status. Thus, it has been found in this vulnerable immobile group that there is an increased number of long bone fractures.

Optimizing nutritional status, appropriate exposure to sunlight to promote vitamin D absorption, appropriate dietetic supplements and the avoidance of some medications such as anticonvulsants that can have an adverse effect on bone density are all useful prophylactically. Some specific treatments can also be used. These include particularly the use of biphosphonates.

The subject has been well reviewed by Houlihan and Stevenson (2009).

Epilepsy
The prevalence of epilepsy, best defined as recurrent seizures, is much higher in people with CP and other neurodisabilities than in the general population. Epilepsy in CP is secondary, that is it is symptomatic and occurs as a consequence of the brain damage that has caused the motor disorder and other impairments. For the large majority of

people with CP who have epilepsy, their seizure disorder is not especially intrusive and may consist of relatively brief and infrequent episodes that, if need be, can be kept under control with appropriate anticonvulsant therapy. In a small minority, however – and this is particularly the case for young children who have evidence of extensive brain damage – their epilepsy can be both severe and relatively refractory to treatment.

The principles of management are the same as those that apply when epilepsy presents in the otherwise unimpaired population. These consist of confirmation of the diagnosis from observation and investigation if at all possible, the thoughtful use of relevant anticonvulsant therapy and consideration for those who have very refractory seizures of other treatment approaches including the ketogenic diet, vagal nerve stimulation and, in specific circumstances, neurosurgical interventions.

The possible side effects of anticonvulsant therapy always need to be kept in mind, especially in children and adults who have communication impairments. Untoward effects that include overall depression of functioning in people with CP are well recognized.

Resources for interventions

A major challenge for parents of children with CP is to find appropriate intervention services and to evaluate the validity of the claims that are made about those services. Information is available from a myriad of sources – professionals, other parents, the web, parent and professional magazines, the popular press, the opinions of friends and family, etc. It can be challenging for parents (and indeed for professionals) to separate wheat from chaff among the often elaborate claims that may be made about the effectiveness of some treatments. This is particularly true of for-profit interventions that are advertised and sold on the Internet or in parent magazines and that make claims which seem exaggerated. We advise that a 'buyer beware' attitude is a sensible approach in these situations.

As we have emphasized throughout the book, the first essential step regarding any intervention is to decide on the goals of treatment. Goals should be set collaboratively by parents and therapists, and should, in our opinion, be directed at the achievement of functionally useful outcomes that address activities and participation (Ketelaar et al. 2001). The laudable but vague goal to 'improve function' should be broken down into measurable steps, so that the effectiveness of treatment can be evaluated against those goals. And, of course, the 'steps' should be meaningful to the child and family. A recent handbook by Dodd et al. (2010) provides excellent examples of how this approach can be implemented in practice.

We have discussed elsewhere the need for a critical appraisal of any interventions that are being offered to children (see Chapter 6). We value the logic of the WHO's ICF (World Health Organization 2001) (see Chapter 7). When applying this approach to any health condition, it is important to identify where the targets of proposed interventions for a child with CP fit in the framework, and to seek evidence that the intervention is likely to 'work' for that purpose and for a child like this. This framework also helps to identify specific activity/participation goals that will enhance the child's functioning, as well as the steps needed to achieve these goals.

Another approach to considering biomedical and technical interventions in CP, proposed by Heinen et al. (2009), aggregates several 'sources of variation' (such as children's age, Gross Motor Function Classification System level and available interventions) into a potentially useful multidimensional approach to decision-making.

The assumptions behind traditional approaches to intervention in CP, whether or not these were stated explicitly, usually involved directing medical treatments or therapy to remediate the biomedical problems (impairments) in body structure and function. There was an implicit belief that in addressing – and where possible 'fixing' – the impairments, one would de facto see changes in functioning. This idea was based on a belief that in CP, problems such as impaired range of motion, or spasticity, were the factors ('causes') limiting people's functional capacity. In this way of thinking, changes to those impairments ought to lead to improvements in functioning.

To date, the limited evidence shows that this idea has not stood up to critical scrutiny and that changes in body structure and function do not necessarily lead to improvements in activity or participation (Wright et al. 2007). Thus, it is important to look for evidence that any potential change in a child's impairment status is likely to affect their functioning, and not simply try to change their 'impairments' in body structure and function with the assumption that function will improve. (It should be added that we also do not know whether changes in people's participation are associated with changes in body structure and function, because those studies remain to be undertaken. The proposition is certainly worth exploring carefully.)

Changing perspectives on development and disability

There are other examples of how an evolution in our understanding of child development, and of disorders in general, has changed how we think about 'treatment' in CP. It has traditionally been thought that 'normal' function was a necessary underpinning for children with CP to achieve milestones and function well, and hence was the desired target outcome. In so far as children with CP almost always have differences and limitations in aspects of function (what some people refer to as 'abnormalities'), it therefore seemed logical that we should try to encourage and promote 'normal' function and prevent children from doing things 'abnormally'. This has led to ideas about what is and is not acceptable.

A favourite example is the proscription against W-sitting. It has traditionally been believed that this posture promoted internal rotation of the hips and would 'cause' later orthopaedic problems. Parents were strongly advised to change their child's position to a side-sitting or tailor (cross-legged) position.

Parents who are honest and trust us report that this is a losing battle that they quickly give up trying to fight, let alone win. This is the case both because children cannot maintain these 'normal' positions and because the W-sitting position is incredibly adaptive for any child who can adopt it. The internally rotated legs, with the feet lateral to the vertical axis of the body, work the way outriggers do on a Hawaiian canoe, or training wheels do on a young child's two-wheel bicycle: they provide lateral postural stability for children that allows them to maintain a straight back and have two hands free for play – both of which are achievements that are rarely possible with side-sitting or other prescribed positions.

It is also important to comment again on the ICF ideas about the importance of promoting 'activities' that enable 'participation' to happen. A child with CP who is prevented from sitting independently on the floor cannot as easily and comfortably experience the activity of sitting for play. This in turn potentially limits their capacity to participate in play. Given that we currently have no way to 'fix' internally rotated hips to prevent W-sitting, and in light of the ICF ideas about functional achievement, it seems logical to 'allow' (we would say encourage) children to be individually adaptive to the ways their bodies work, in the service of functional achievement, even if there is a trade-off with 'normality'.

(As for whether W-sitting leads to later orthopaedic difficulties, we are aware of no prospective longitudinal studies that have established this connection, let alone a causal pathway. And we like to remind people that any child who can W-sit already has increased capacity for internal rotation of their hips – that is what makes this position possible and comfortable for them.)

Therapy in practice

In summary, this chapter reminds us that the general health and well-being of children with CP need to be considered carefully. We argue that it is important that the people who work with families of children with CP have experience and expertise. Special attention is needed to address the common health challenges to which people with CP are at increased risk, and to consider opportunities for preventative initiatives that address, in particular, nutritional status and bone health. The following chapter discusses more specifically principles and issues of 'therapy' and 'management' of children with CP.

References

Brooks J, Day S, Shavelle R, Strauss D (2011) Low weight, morbidity, and mortality in children with cerebral palsy: new clinical growth charts. *Pediatrics* 128: e299–307.

Day SM, Strauss DJ, Vachon PJ, Rosenbloom L, Shavelle RM, Wu YW (2007) Growth patterns in a population of children and adolescents with cerebral palsy. *Dev Med Child Neurol* 49: 167–7

Dodd K, Imms C, Taylor NF (2010) *Physiotherapy and Occupational Therapy for People with Cerebral Palsy: A Problem-Based Approach to Assessment and Management.* London: Mac Keith Press.

Heinen F, Schröder AS, Döderlein L et al. (2009) Grafikgestützter Konsensus für die Behandlung von Bewegungsstörungen bei Kindern mit bilateralen spastischen Zerebralparesen (BS-CP). Graphically based consensus on the treatment of movement disorders in children with bilateral spastic cerebral palsy (BS-CP). Therapiekurven – CP-Motorik Motor treatment curves in CP. *Monatsschr Kinderheilkd* 157: 789–94.

Houlihan CM, Stevenson RD (2009) Bone density in cerebral palsy. *Phys Med Rehabil Clin* 20: 493–508.

Ketelaar M, Vermeer A, Hart H, van Petegem-van Beek E, Helders PJ (2001) Effects of a functional therapy program on motor abilities of children with cerebral palsy. *Phys Ther* 81: 1534–45.

Odman P, Oberg B (2005) Effectiveness of intensive training for children with cerebral palsy – a comparison between child and youth rehabilitation and conductive education. *J Rehabil Med* 37: 263–70.

Rosenbaum P (2009) Putting child development back into developmental disabilities. *Dev Med Child Neurol* 51: 251.

Strauss D, Cable W, Shavelle R (1999) Causes of excess mortality in cerebral palsy. *Dev Med Child Neurol* 41: 580–5.

Sullivan P (2009) *Feeding and Nutrition in Children with Neurodevelopmental Disability.* London: Mac Keith Press.

Wright FV, Rosenbaum PL, Fehlings D (2007) How do changes in impairment, activity, and participation relate to each other? Study of children with cerebral palsy (CP) who have received lower extremity botulinum toxin type-A (Bt-A) injections. *Dev Med Child Neurol* 50: 283–9.

World Health Organization (2001) *International Classification of Functioning, Disability and Health (ICF).* Geneva: World Health Organization.

Chapter 12

Therapists and therapies in cerebral palsy

with Margaret Mayston

Overview

Therapists are trained professionals with a range of skills and knowledge about the workings of the human body, with a special emphasis on aspects of human functioning. People who work with disabled children are sometimes referred to as 'developmental' therapists in order to recognize the importance of their understanding of the ways that disabilities may impact on children's development. 'Occupational therapists' use and adapt everyday activities to promote health and well-being (World Federation of Occupational Therapists 2011). 'Physical therapists' have advanced understanding of how the body moves and what keeps it from moving well, and they use this to promote wellness, mobility and independence (World Confederation for Physical Therapy 2011). Therapists who focus on communication are known as 'speech–language therapists' (or speech–language 'pathologists'). In reality, therapists with these specific skills will have some overlap with each other as they all aim to help children to optimize their participation in all aspects of daily life. While these are the most frequently recognized professional groupings in childhood disability, there are many other 'therapists', who often focus on particular activities such as music, horseback riding, swimming and so on.

There are many therapy options available for people with cerebral palsy (CP), and the number increases as new ideas, knowledge and evidence emerge. Unfortunately, as yet there are few answers as to what works best, at what age/stage and how. It is also difficult to be prescriptive because each child and family is individual and may have different needs. Studies are needed to show us what strategies work best, for whom, and how and why it is that they are effective. This chapter does not have the scope to cover details or to mention every type of therapy or adjunctive treatment available, but hopefully it provides an overview of important principles for the therapy and management of CP.

Therapies and therapists: principles and perspectives

Therapy is considered an integral element of the management of people with CP. Despite this reality, there have been few systematic evaluations of the various available therapies as to their efficacy, theoretical basis or whether one is better than another (see Mayston [2004] for a review of therapy approaches). A review of controlled trials published by Anttila et al. (2008) found limited evidence supporting the use of hand therapy and hippotherapy, but these, like many therapy studies, were trials carried out with only a small number of participants. The relevance of the evidence presented in these studies is complicated by the fact that therapists often use an eclectic approach with mixed strategies from different therapy systems. This of course makes evaluation of any particular system of therapy almost impossible. For the family of a person with CP, it is then difficult to know what is the best therapy for their individual situation. The Internet provides a large range of options; unfortunately for the uninformed consumer, one often finds unsubstantiated claims made by people whose skills and qualifications are usually of uncertain value (Rosenbaum 2003; Mayston 2004). These challenges are discussed briefly at the end of this chapter.

What is therapy?

Perhaps this is a good place to consider what we mean by therapy. Can we define it? Most people probably think that therapy is what is done to and with the child by a therapist, and/or view it as a set of exercises; however, it is better to think of therapy as a process of helping a family (and a child) to learn ways for a child to function optimally in their many environments. It is not simply a matter of having as much therapy as possible, but rather involves using the therapist's expertise to explore ways that will enable the child and the family to live as fully and functionally as possible. In terms of the International Classification of Functioning, Disability and Health (ICF) (see Chapter 7), we want to promote optimal participation in daily life by enhancing activities and minimizing residual impairments such as musculoskeletal and cognitive limitations that are recognized aspects of CP (Rosenbaum et al. 2007; Rosenbaum and Gorter 2011). It is accepted that CP cannot be cured, but its effects *can* be modified, and we all need to be aware – both professionals and clients (i.e. the child and family) – of what is possible and what is not so that a realistic approach to management is taken.

Therapy traditions

It is appropriate to open the discussion of therapies with a word about the so-called 'traditional therapies' that have long been the mainstay of intervention in the twentieth century (see Mayston [2004] for a review).

The best known traditional therapies are Bobath therapy (also known as neurodevelopmental therapy or NDT), and conductive education (CE). Both are practised worldwide and Bobath/NDT in particular offers training courses in their philosophy and practice to professionals, which has ensured its continued strong presence in the favoured therapy listing. Bobath therapy changed the direction of management of children with CP in the middle of the last century owing to the recognition of what we now understand as neuroplasticity – the ability of the brain to alter its structure and function according to the experiences it is afforded. Bobath focused on tone and postural activity as the main body structure and function 'impairment' factors underpinning function (now referred to as activity and participation). While Bobath/NDT made an enormous contribution to the progress of CP management, there is no robust evidence to support its efficacy, and because different practitioners worldwide practise it in different ways it is hard to define exactly what it is today (Butler and Darrah 2001; Mayston 2008).

The second well-known therapy approach for children with CP, CE (Bourke-Taylor et al. 2007), was never meant to be a therapy system, although it is viewed as one in some countries but as a complementary/alternative therapy in others. The ideas behind this approach to the management of children with CP are based on principles of good pedagogy that are not unique to CE. Underlying CE are the notions that there is value in working with children in groups, and that facilitating children's activities by having them say what they are doing and do what they are saying promotes learning. There are many sensible ideas within the CE approach, although there is no evidence that CE produces better outcomes than other approaches (Darrah et al. 2004; Oldman and Oberg 2005; Tuersley-Dixon and Frederickson 2010).

Both of these schools of therapy have something to offer, but it is unlikely that either can offer the complete package to any individual. We all need to be able to underpin our decision-making with a balanced view of the biomedical and psychosocial needs of each child and family. To do this might require us to take a step back, review the available neuroscience, physiology, evidence and intervention options, and on that basis advise and provide what is needed to optimize the child's participation. Such a stance may mean discarding long-held beliefs (Damiano 2006) and a refocusing of therapeutic efforts.

We would add that it is beyond the scope of this book to detail and comment on the wide range of educational hypotheses, approaches and systems that are applied to children with neurological disabilities and other special educational needs. Rather, reference should be made to relevant texts. We would emphasize, however, that the principles of providing relevant inputs and promoting access to these are the same as when therapy for children with CP is considered.

Basic ingredients of therapy for children with cerebral palsy: an approach to the issues

We are aware of an increasingly wide range of therapy options, but it is evident that no one system will provide the complete package. Therefore, what we have tried to present in this chapter are the essential points to bear in mind when making therapy choices.

Many questions remain unanswered, such as when therapy should start, how long it should last, how often it should be provided and so on. Although no long-term studies of outcomes for these children give clear answers to these questions, we can probably identify key stages of development when the focus of intervention needs to change to adapt to the child's changing capacities and developmental tasks. It might be helpful to identify some guiding principles for therapy intervention, many of which will already be apparent, before considering some of the specific types of evidence-based intervention.

Professionals working in the management of CP need to be experts in the field and have a good understanding of all aspects of typical child development, and of course the multifaceted nature of CP at all stages of the lifespan. Table 12.1 shows the key elements of gross motor functioning throughout the lifespan, which may provide a general guide for the focus of intervention at any particular age. Readers should also refer to the motor development curves for the Gross Motor Function Classification System (GMFCS) levels (Appendix V), which also provide a rough guide to ultimate motor outcomes and times of developmental plateau (Rosenbaum et al. 2002).

The following key concepts should serve to guide all therapeutic interventions for children with developmental disabilities:

- Clear goal setting is essential, in partnership with the child and family, and with clearly defined participation goal(s).

- Goals should take into account all aspects of the child/family's activity/participation, for example play, school, social, fitness; this requires input from the team members working with the family. Goals need to be specific, relevant and measurable, as well as time limited.

- Measurement of activity/participation and *regular* review of these measures is important, with revision of goals as changes occur or the goals become dated.

- Engagement of the child/family in the therapy programme is vital. Ensure that the child and family know what they are doing and why those activities have been identified. Team members need to provide clear instruction, training and reminders as appropriate to enable successful engagement in the programme.

- Clear strategies should be provided that can be confidently practised by the child and family during daily life.

- Therapists should offer advice about the provision of splints, aids, appliances and adjuncts and should review these recommendations regularly as the child grows and changes.

- There are no formulae or recipes for intervention. Therapy must be tailored to the individual's needs and abilities (strengths), and, in our view, be consistent with developmental and functional goals and not simply address 'impairments' at the biomedical level of body structure and function.

Table 12.1 A lifespan view of general therapy goal areas

Age range	Focus of development at this stage	Therapy focus for GMFCS I–III	For GMFCS IV and V consider in addition:
Neonatal period	Adaptation to extrauterine environment	Early intervention with focus on caregiver–child interaction/bond. Creating the appropriate environment and ways of engagement with the infant, daily life handling/holding, caring for the infant. For the extremely preterm infant, there is a need to minimize sensory experiences and handling, as preterm infants are unable to tolerate even usual levels of stimulation, e.g. touch, noise, light, etc. Early challenges with feeding may be the first sign of a problem	High likelihood of seizures, visual impairment and need for a feeding tube. Assist parents to come to terms with the complexity of their situation
Early (~0–8mo)	Self-discovery and communication	Awareness of self, the other and discovery of own body enabled by midline orientation and self-exploration, especially early attention to hand functioning. Differentiation of cries and early communication by varied sounds/facial expressions/gestures and body movement. Developing a reference point for interaction with the external world. Early floor mobility (rolling, pivoting) and experiences of different postures, e.g. prone, sitting	Provision of assistive devices – good, supportive seating and mobility (car seat, pushchair, etc.). Hip surveillance will become highly important. Participate in group programmes, music/movement, etc.

Age range	Focus of development at this stage	Therapy focus for GMFCS I–III	For GMFCS IV and V consider in addition:
8–20mo	Early floor mobility and exploration	Many ways of moving on the floor to enable discovery of the self with respect to others and the environment. Likes/dislikes; cause/effect. Mobility and exploration mediate learning. Introduce early communication with gestures, signs, simple pictures; self-feeding. Begin to monitor musculoskeletal status and provide aids/orthoses as appropriate	Consider use of assisted power mobility to enable exploration. Monitor positioning for eating/drinking, check for reflux
Toddler (20–36mo)	Mobility and peers	Realization that one is not the centre of the world and needs to interact with others. Provide alternative means of mobility as needed with supportive equipment to enable upright postures and participation in the world. Continue communication/musculoskeletal management as needed (this is ongoing through all life stages). Behavioural: needs to learn boundaries like any typically developing child	Children at GMFCS level V achieve 90% of their motor development by age 3, so future management plans can be formulated at this stage. Independent walking is not an option. Consideration of mobility options

Table 12.1 Continued

Age range	Focus of development at this stage	Therapy focus for GMFCS I–III	For GMFCS IV and V consider in addition:
Nursery school (3–5y)	Need to fit a structure; peer interaction	Required to fit in with group activities and attend as needed. Often requires a reliable floor sitting position: needs to develop a variety of ways of doing activities, e.g. sitting postures/standing/ mobility. Importance of work on standing for later standing transfers if at all possible	Children in GMFCS level IV have achieved 90% of their motor development by age 3y 6mo and future management plans can be set out now. Introduce technology early – this will be important for the future. Switching, etc.
School years (6–11y)	Independence in and outside the classroom	Mobility in and outside the classroom and independence at recreational times, making friends – acceptance. Hip surveillance always very important (in GMFCS levels III–V) but more so at this stage as more time spent sitting and greater mobility demands to keep up with the group. Recreational/physical activities important	Positioning, transfers and musculoskeletal management are to the fore. Hoisting may be started and this requires good caregiver training about risk assessment

Age range	Focus of development at this stage	Therapy focus for GMFCS I–III	For GMFCS IV and V consider in addition:
Puberty (~12y)	Growth spurt: mobility challenge/ decisions	Important transition to secondary school and further development of independence and choice. Early mobility options may need to be questioned, and will be again in the future. Another critical time for musculoskeletal system, especially for muscle/ joint contractures due to rapid skeletal growth. Develop recreational/sports activities	Surgical intervention may be necessary to enable optimal positioning in sitting as standing devices which are useful to maintain musculoskeletal integrity may be discontinued by many
Adolescence (12–18y)	Social participation; sexuality; relationships; occupation; maintain physical level	Focus on scholastic achievement and making meaningful friendships; higher education; getting ready for living away from home. Independence in all aspects. Psychosocial well-being: 'talking therapies' may be of value at this time and onwards. Continue with recreational activities to maintain fitness and contribute to well-being. Specific therapeutic input as needed	Spinal surgery may be indicated for scoliosis. Monitor health and well-being. Particular emphasis on caregiver well-being and support
Adult	Occupation; independence; relationships; 'wear and tear'	Maintaining useful and fulfilling employment; relationships; child bearing. May require specific focused physical surveillance and intervention for pain, joint wear and tear and general mobility in addition to fitness/ recreational activities	Ongoing surveillance and caregiver support

GMFCS, Gross Motor Function Classification System.

It goes without saying that to apply these basic principles requires a thorough assessment, analysis and interpretation of the child's activity/participation, and an understanding of contextual factors such as their family dynamics, attitudes, socioeconomic situation and parents' aspirations for their child. There is also a need for forward thinking on the basis of the therapists' knowledge of the natural course of the effects of CP according to age and type of CP, and implications for the future. Three broad areas of challenge for the person with CP impact on their ability to participate in life: mobility, communication and use of the hands for self-care and all tasks involving manipulation and support. Most parents consider that the ultimate goal is 'that my child will walk'; the question of whether this will happen, and when, is the one most often asked of the therapist. But should this be the ultimate goal?

It may be that the ability to use one's arms/hands for support when transferring from bed to wheelchair and to manipulate objects in daily life will facilitate greater independence than an ability to walk between two locations. Consider, for example, a child with CP in GMFCS level III who can manage to walk between the car and classroom, to the toilet, to the meal table, but is unable to do anything once she arrives there. She is unable to use her upper limbs for support or manipulation, making her reliant on others for mealtime assistance and for all other activities of daily life. Upper limb functioning seems to be the key to independence, and although it is often thought to be the domain of the occupational therapist, all team members should be integrating this into their goals. For example, the physiotherapist can advise on transfers and the use of walking aids; the speech and language therapist can address self-feeding and use of communication aids; the occupational therapist can look at dressing and writing skills; the teacher can explore how these abilities are integrated into classroom activities and accommodated as needed; and the physical education instructor can focus on exercise and fitness activities, to name a few of the possible contributions to promoting independence.

Balancing biomechanics and neuronal functioning

Every physiology text shows us that muscles generate optimal forces when in a mid-position. Very often, however, children with CP have muscle imbalances and joint limitations that can impede their ability to produce sufficient force to carry out everyday activities easily, or at all. As the child with CP grows, muscle growth does not match bone growth, and these imbalances can become more evident with time. In these circumstances, the challenge is to minimize or prevent such limitations from becoming fixed, because the imbalances can become almost impossible to manage effectively. Very often the use of splints, medication and surgery will be necessary.

Passive movements/stretches have been a mainstay of traditional physiotherapy and occupational therapy and yet there is no evidence to support their use (Pin et al. 2006; Harvey et al. 2007). Limited evidence suggests that the amount of time needed to stretch a muscle to maintain its length is several hours per day (Tardieu et al. 1988), which rules out the use of manual stretching and will necessitate the use of aids/appliances if it is to be used at all.

The need for an activity-based therapy

In the previous chapter, we indicated that neuroplasticity is the basis of change in the nervous system, and that it can either help or hinder developmental progress. It is clear from the literature that positive adaptive changes are driven by activities that are relevant to the person and are appropriately challenging, but not too difficult. This means that the goals we set need to be meaningful to the individual, achievable and practised often enough to drive these changes. Currently there are no good answers to the question of 'How long must I practise to drive this change?' (Note that this same question might be asked by parents of any child learning to play a musical instrument.) The evidence suggests that all therapy needs to be activity based to optimize the opportunities for brain adaptation and learning, and that adjunctive interventions such as the use of splints, anti-spasticity medication and surgery also require activity-based therapy to optimize their effects (Harvey 2010). 'Activity' means that the child is an active participant in the therapy – whether it be an impairment-based treatment like practising a task component such as grasp and release to enable more effective play or dressing, or whether it is the whole task activity of play or dressing.

Meaningful tasks are essential to any therapy activity, and, as has been emphasized in this book, approaches that are task focused have been shown to result in positive outcomes (Ketelaar et al. 2001). Practice of tasks can be made easier by certain therapy strategies such as organizing the environment to promote practice (Darrah et al. 2011) or providing equipment, splints, aids and appliances. Specific therapeutic handling to optimize muscle length for best activation to support an activity, or to practise task components, can also be useful and is discussed in the next section of this chapter. These factors are relevant for all areas of intervention: mobility, communication, hand functioning and the practice of all daily tasks including family/peer interactions, education, occupation and leisure.

A few general principles about the *content* of a therapy programme will be discussed before we talk about some specific interventions for which there is a good body of evidence, albeit on small numbers of participants and generally on children at GMFCS levels I–III. The work of *CanChild* (www.canchild.ca) has produced many useful outcome measures, including the functional way of classifying children with CP with the GMFCS (Palisano et al. 1997, 2008) (see Appendix I). The GMFCS is made up of five levels, is based on a person's ability to self-initiate activities related to sitting and walking, and is also subdivided according to age.

We also need to define what constitutes 'treatment' and what constitutes 'management'. Treatment is best viewed as the application of a specific intervention, whether it be task practice, handling by the therapist/caregiver or use of equipment, surgery, medication or splints, to name a few. Management is generally thought of as a broader concept that involves taking an overall view of the child's situation and ensuring that all aspects of their CP are taken into account in their therapy programme. The decision to focus more on treatment or management may also depend in part on the child's GMFCS level (as described by Dodd et al. 2010). For example, a child at GMFCS level V may have significant motor impairment but above-average cognitive functioning; postural management, transfers and powered mobility will be key elements of their treatment. But in terms of this child's participation, attention also needs to be given to their access to technology for learning, communication, education and ultimately for occupation; architectural barriers may need to be addressed as well. Management implies looking at the child's day from a 24-hour perspective and ensuring that all aspects of their life are being given appropriate attention and intervention, hence the need to integrate therapy into the total management package and to appreciate the contribution of the many team members. We provide treatment to achieve management in order to enhance function and life quality.

There is much discussion about whether therapy should include hands-on strategies, and currently there are no experimental studies that can answer this question conclusively; however, the child's GMFCS level will be an important factor in making this decision (Mayston 2007). The ideas below are predominantly based on clinical experience along with some available literature that leads us to suggest the following guiding principles, which need to be applied according to the child's GMFCS level, environment and cultural context.

- Any therapy programme should consider the whole child – this may require input from several team members, so all need to speak the same language and agree on participation goals.

- Engagement with the family and child is an essential starting point – this means understanding the family context and engaging the child in play and daily life activities to determine if, what and how specific impairments need to be addressed, and what will be the relevant activity and participation goals to set and practise. A good guide to goal setting can come from knowing what the child is about to learn to do, can do with a little assistance and/or what the parents (and child) perceive as the next step in their development.

- All systems need to be in their optimal state to enable effective activity practice. This includes sensory, motor, cognitive, perceptual and biomechanical systems. Sensory systems are essential for controlling movements and for learning – we learn the sensation of a task. For example, perception is critical for safe, enjoyable movement in space and for the ability to identify objects. From a cognitive perspective, a child needs to be able to engage in the task and understand its relevance, and also have opportunities to solve problems relating to the task as this promotes learning. We need to refrain from telling the child what to do all the time.

- A specific point perhaps needs to be made about the biomechanical factors underling task performance. Muscles need to be long enough and strong enough to effect movements. This may require 'hands-on' or other techniques such as positioning, progressive strength training and the use of adjunctive treatments such as splints and pharmacological agents. Handling and positioning are the mainstays of the physical techniques that therapists use to give the child the possibility to engage successfully in daily activities (Dodd et al. 2010). Handling can help the child to learn the idea of a movement to be practised, or can elongate their muscles to enable the movement to be practised more easily. These handling techniques can be used within daily tasks. One example is the use of handling to maintain appropriate alignment of the head and neck to make it possible for the child to swallow more safely; another is elongation and activation of hip and knee flexors in the prone or supine position, or in a standing frame, to enable easier standing practice. A child may learn to stretch their own muscles by weight-bearing; for example, a child with weakness and stiffness on one side can be taught to take weight through their arm in sitting or standing during dressing/undressing or during other tasks to ensure that their arm is not always held in a shortened position, which can result in permanent muscle shortening. There are many other examples, some of which are given by Dodd et al. (2010) (see Chapter 4) as well as Finnie (see Bower 2009).

- If handling techniques are used by the therapist, these must be simple and easy for the child and family to learn so that they can be used within task practice at home, and by anyone in the child's many environments, particularly at school. Handling has its place, but it is absolutely essential to realize that handling is not therapy when used alone or used passively, or if used continuously. 'Hands on' is only a therapy technique and not a treatment in itself, and is only appropriate when used in conjunction with active practice which has the intention of enabling 'hands off' as the child learns to do the activity on their own. Handling is about enabling, and this point cannot be overemphasized.

- It should be clear that if tasks are to be learned, they need to be practised, so everyone needs to know how to practise effectively. The practice activities are not exercises but ways of carrying out all daily life activities, hence the need to learn the how and why of handling and positioning, active practice and the how and why of equipment use (e.g. standing frames and special seating) and splints as needed. Handling and positioning are especially relevant to children at GMFCS levels III–V (particularly GMFCS IV and V) but may also be used in some cases for children at GMFCS levels I and II.

- Progress needs to be monitored, therefore regular measures against preset goals, reviews and updates are needed.

All therapy should focus on activity and participation, even if there are elements of intervention at an impairment level as part of that approach. Most of the known therapies, including the named approaches, would claim to be activity based, but some therapies, such as 'constraint therapy', treadmill training and task training, are obviously significantly more activity focused. These are discussed briefly below. Although muscle strengthening is an impairment-level intervention, discussion about it is also included, as it has been neglected in therapy programmes until recently.

Thus, one therapy that has emerged in recent years is constraint-induced movement therapy (CIMT; Taub et al. 2004). This therapy has a sound experimental basis in the animal literature (Nudo et al. 1996) and in studies of adults following a stroke (Liepert et al. 2000; Wolf et al. 2008). The studies show that for a person with hemiplegia and some ability to use their affected hand, restraint of the less affected side for a recommended 6 hours per day for 2 weeks can improve hand function in the impaired side such that it can be used with greater frequency and skill in daily life activities. There have been a few small studies on children with CP using a modified approach (Eliasson et al. 2005; Naylor and Bower, 2005; Aarts et al. 2010). It is possible that this approach could be used in a group setting (as in the study by Aarts et al. 2010) to enable several children to benefit and also to promote social and peer interaction.

There are two notes of caution when considering this approach. First, CIMT is thought to be detrimental for very young infants (age <12mo) with hemiplegia because it may impair the further development of unaffected areas of the central nervous system – in this case the surviving corticospinal tract from the intact hemisphere (Salimi et al. 2008). Second, it seems that CIMT might be more effective if combined with bimanual training (Aarts et al. 2010). It is not yet clear whether bimanual training might even be as effective as CIMT in some circumstances (Gordon et al. 2008; Boyd et al. 2010), but studies are currently investigating this question. Clinical experience suggests that a modified version of CIMT can also be applied to children with asymmetrical total body involvement when one side functions very much better than the other. It is really all about focusing on the activity of the more affected side to enable two sides to work together more effectively.

Treadmill training is another intervention with a sound theoretical basis and is also a 'task-focused' activity. As yet there is no robust experimental evidence to support its use clinically, although there are some promising studies that will be mentioned. There is solid evidence from the animal literature that networks of neurons in the lumbar region of the spinal cord generate rhythmical locomotor (walking) activity (Bélanger et al. 1996). These do not need the brain to activate them, although it is necessary that the brain influences these networks to enable adaptation of the basic programme to all environmental demands. We must also keep in mind that walking requires internally generated postural control, and if this is lacking then external assistance may be needed to enable functional use of the locomotor pattern.

Thus, the promotion of stepping activity needs to be kept in the context of the child's capacity and performance. This scientific knowledge forms the basis of treadmill training with partial body weight support, which is predominantly used for people with spinal cord injury and stroke, but which has also been tested for children with CP at all GMFCS levels (Schindl et al. 2000; Dodd and Foley 2007; Willoughby et al. 2010). A recent review (Willoughby et al. 2009) has suggested that this therapy modality is safe and feasible for children with CP to train in walking and improve walking speed (Dodd and Foley 2007), but the effects are not yet well enough researched or conclusive to be able to recommend it for all types of CP (see review by Mutlu et al. 2009; Willoughby et al. 2010). There may also be other benefits from this type of intervention, such as changes in muscle strength, positive effects on bone density, ease of wheelchair transfers (Schindl et al. 2000) and improved fitness (Blundell et al. 2003). Treadmill training also offers the possibility of being an 'inclusive' activity as many people go to the fitness centre and participate in treadmill training to promote general fitness and aerobic capacity. This kind of 'therapy' could also provide an opportunity for family and peer activities.

There is little doubt that for many children muscle strengthening should be undertaken, as it is now clear that muscle weakness is a significant impairment for children with CP. Promotion of muscle strengthening has been lacking in traditional therapy approaches and has recently become more prominent in the therapy toolbox. Although several reviews advocate its effectiveness in improving muscle strength and scores on the Gross Motor Function Measure (GMFM) (Damiano and Abel 1998; Dodd et al. 2002), this intervention, like all others, has different effects on different children and may not always be of benefit (Damiano et al. 2010).

It is also important to bear in mind that some studies have shown that improvements in strength are not always accompanied by improvements in mobility (Scholtes et al. 2010). It is possible that interventions like this at an impairment level may also require an activity-based intervention to maximize their effect. Alternatively, muscles can be loaded during a functional task, as shown in the study by Liao et al. (2007) when a weighted backpack was applied to a sitting to standing task. A task approach gives some meaning to the person, and so they are more likely to enjoy it and therefore to practise it sufficiently to induce positive change. While this is an impairment-based intervention, it is also another means of inclusive activity that can be carried out at the local community fitness centre (if the appropriate insurance cover is in place for younger people). Several studies have reported positive benefits for adolescents and young adults (Taylor et al. 2004). This type of intervention may be more appropriate for teenagers and younger and older adults in whom there are no concerns about the developing skeletal system, which seems to be vulnerable to loading in younger children (Faigenbaum 1999).

Mobility
There are many acceptable ways to achieve mobility in the early years, including rolling, crawling and cruising, but very soon upright mobility becomes the norm and often the desired parental goal despite the reality that for many children with CP this evolution will not take place (Bottos and Gericke 2003; Palisano et al. 2010). Because GMFCS levels are effectively stable in individual children and adolescents, they are a useful predictor of gross motor functioning and thus enable us to predict the possible future mobility outcome for a child with CP. A study of a large number of children with CP using the GMFM (Russell et al. 1989) showed that it was possible to predict future mobility and gross motor function according to GMFCS level (Rosenbaum et al. 2002; see Appendix V). These data provide a sound basis to facilitate realistic discussions of future mobility options.

Each person requires careful evaluation, and mobility performance and aids need to be monitored. Is the walking aid one that the child can operate independently, or does it require that the child be placed in it? While such walkers give the child early upright mobility experience and a means to explore, it is very doubtful that they will serve as a long-term option. Powered mobility including the use of sit/stand chairs is increasingly chosen by young people with CP with limited walking ability and can also be useful in maintaining musculoskeletal integrity as well as making possible easier access to higher surfaces. It should be noted here that an ability to take weight in standing to enable assistance with standing transfers (as can often be possible in people at GMFCS levels III or IV) is an important element of independence. Thus, if possible, the ability to stand and to achieve standing transfers should be maintained. A realistic approach to the use of assisted standing and taking a few steps in therapy programmes clearly requires some review and thought, because although this ability may not translate into fully independent mobility, it can have powerful impacts on carers and on functional capacity.

Aids to mobility take many forms, for example walking and wheeled and powered mobility devices, and an individual may require more than one of these aids depending on their level of activity. The Functional Mobility Scale is a useful way of determining mobility needs (Graham et al. 2004). Whatever device is chosen, it needs to be appropriate for the size and strength of the child, their environment (accessibility), and their level of functioning, and it should be introduced early to provide a means of exploration and participation as well as a sense of empowerment and a positive effect on the family (Butler et al. 1983, Butler 1986; Tefft et al. 2011).

Adjunctive interventions

The musculoskeletal system is the effector system which makes our actions happen, and it needs to function adequately to enable effective muscle force generation through sufficient joint range to allow participation in daily life activities including mobility. One of the greatest challenges facing physical therapists is the management of the musculoskeletal system to counteract and minimize contractures and deformities, and this can become a significant concern for parents and their children, particularly at times of rapid growth when the muscle does not keep up with the bone. Adjunctive interventions, in the form of splints, pharmacological treatment, equipment and surgery, are an important ingredient of intervention for the musculoskeletal system. These can be prescribed after the use of objective assessments such as gait analysis but in some settings are prescribed on the basis of experience and clinical examination.

It is outside the scope of this book to describe and detail the indications for and the range of orthopaedic procedures that are available and that are currently used for children and adults with CP. These range from those that are used prophylactically, through specific therapeutic interventions to maintain and promote function, to salvage procedures, for example to relieve pain and discomfort. Reference should be made to Horstman and Bleck's (2007) comprehensive text for a detailed consideration of this subject.

In recent years, it has become more common to perform a single-event multilevel surgical procedure to the lower limbs (Graham and Selber 2003). These are preferable to the previous stage-like progression that meant that a child had to take considerable periods of time out of school to undergo procedures almost on an annual basis for several years – the so-called 'birthday surgery' phenomenon. This surgery requires good physiotherapy preparation and postoperative management, and the timing of it is also important to minimize the need for further procedures at a later date (Harvey 2010). Surgery for the upper limbs is less commonly done and is usually undertaken for cosmetic reasons. It is more usual to use a focal pharmacological agent like botulinum toxin (BoNT-A) in these situations, usually with specific functional or cosmetic goals in mind (Duncan 2010).

BoNT-A treatment is now one of the mainstays of spasticity management in CP and is often used in the years before surgery is appropriate. It has the advantage of being reversible (thus it can also be a useful indicator for whether or not surgery is appropriate) and targeting specific muscles. It is therefore a treatment for focal rather than generalized spasticity. Decisions about the use of BoNT-A need to be made on an individual basis (Harvey 2010). It is also important to combine these injections with physiotherapy to maximize the effects on range of movement and the child's activity and participation (Desloovere et al. 2007). Naumann et al. (2006) have reviewed the safety and efficacy of BoNT-A after long-term use. The long-term effects of its use in very young children are unknown (Barrett 2011), but it has been used in adults for long periods without any described adverse effects.

Oral medications are frequently prescribed to alter muscle tone. They include baclofen and benzodiazepines. Other medications are used in an attempt to limit drooling, reduce unwanted involuntary movements, provide analgesia and treat seizures. In all cases it is important to be clear about and to preset therapeutic goals, and then to evaluate these carefully in order to have a solid evidence base on which to either continue or stop these interventions.

Another intervention for spasticity and muscle spasm is intrathecal baclofen, which has a generalized effect. It is used to reduce muscle excitability throughout the body and is more likely to be considered when there is severe spasticity. Its use has been shown to have a positive effect on care and comfort, but overall its effects require more research (Delgado et al. 2010; Morton et al. 2011).

A surgical approach to spasticity that has been used intermittently over the last 30 or more years is selective dorsal rhizotomy (Smyth and Peacock 2000; Baker and Graham 2011; Grunt et al. 2011, Tedroff et al. 2011). Again, long-term effects are unknown and the time taken to rehabilitate after this procedure is at least a year. The success of any spasticity/spasm-reducing treatment will depend on how much strength the child has to enable their muscles to be used effectively to take advantage of the procedure.

A wide range of aids and orthoses are available that provide dynamic support, and the reader is referred to Morris and Dias (2007) and the consensus report from the International Society of Prosthetics and Orthotics published by Morris et al. (2009) (see also Morris and Condie, 2009). In general, orthoses are used to prevent or correct musculoskeletal deformities and improve physical functioning, and are typically custom made. Decisions need to be made on an individual basis about what type should be used, when it should be worn and for how long. Therapists need to ensure that splints and orthoses – indeed all equipment – are maintained, of good fit and replaced as needed according to size and level of functioning.

Communication

The ability to give a simple and consistent yes/no response can change the world for a person with limited oral communication capacity. Assessment of communication abilities in children with CP is an integral component of their evaluation, and we support the use of measures such as the recently developed Communication Function Classification System (Hidecker et al. 2011). The ideas discussed regarding the provision of mobility aids to enable participation and empowerment also apply to communication. Children with a limited ability to produce words may still be able to use other means: crying, gesture, signs, body movements, subtle behaviours, etc. The use of an augmented communication system needs to be started early, whether via signing, a communication board using real objects or photographs of known objects (e.g. family members, bed, food, etc.), picture exchange communication symbols or technology-based systems. Children at any GMFCS level may have difficulty with oral communication skills. For all children with this type of communication activity limitation, technology can enable very effective means of communicating with others, including the use of cell phones and SMS text messaging.

Clinical experience shows that some children will use mass body patterns – especially mass extension – to communicate that they want attention and/or to indicate their needs, or perhaps to indicate discomfort associated with reflux. Too often therapists interpret this as a dystonic spasm, yet providing a simple way to indicate a yes/no answer may be all that is needed to stop these unnecessary movements and to take away the child's frustration. Although parents are very good at interpreting their child's needs via non-verbal means, sounds and behaviours, communication requires all the people we encounter to understand us, and so when systems are put in place it is important that everyone in the child's life consistently uses the chosen method.

The oromotor activity required for communication is also related to eating and drinking. How the oromotor system is used to manage different textures and types of foods also trains the oromotor system to enable the ability to use speech for communication if applicable for that child. Early eating and drinking patterns and skills can be an indicator of gross oromotor problems. Therapists also need to be aware of signs that the child may be aspirating, for example coughing, choking or voice changes during/after mealtime. Effective and safe eating is essential to ensure adequate nutrition and growth (see Sullivan 2009).

Hand function

The ability to use one's hands for everyday tasks and occupations, or to use a communication or other device, is critical. It is of little value to be able to walk to the toilet, dinner table or desk unless something useful can be done when one gets there. It is impossible to dress and care for oneself without the ability to use our hands. The dependence on the corticospinal tract for discrete finger movements is well known, and yet the corticospinal tract is often damaged or aberrant in children with CP (Carr et al. 1993; Eyre et al. 2007). Beyond that, use of the hands requires a trunk and base of support from the lower limbs to enable movement in space and adequate muscle strength to enable grasp and manipulation of objects. The sensory control of all our activities, but especially our hand activities, is critical. For example, how do you know what is in your pocket if you cannot feel it?

The use of the Manual Ability Classification System (Appendix II) can be helpful when planning the degree of support that is required to enable children to achieve fine motor activities within the home and the school environment (Eliasson et al. 2006).

Maximizing hand function is often seen as the domain of the occupational therapist, and yet it is integral to most activities that the child does and so must be the concern of most of the team members. These activities include finger pointing for communication, holding and manoeuvring a walking aid, work at school, recreational and computer games, etc.

Postural management

An integral component of therapy is postural management, which underlies all the specific therapies and aspects of therapy mentioned so far. It deserves a special mention here as postural management needs to be a part of every aspect of the child's functioning. This will include consideration of positioning for play, school and work, use of orthotics, splints and equipment, sleeping position and providing a sleep system if appropriate. Indeed, as the title implies, it means looking at all aspects of the daily schedule with special reference to postural alignment and activity (see a recent consensus statement on postural management by Gericke 2006).

Each child will require a different individualized mix of ingredients on their pathway to optimal participation in life, and these will vary at different ages and stages. For example, a child at puberty undergoing a growth spurt may need more focused input to maintain joint range to enable effective muscle action. This also means that we should realize that at certain times maintenance of activity/participation level is a valid goal and represents 'success', and that progress in terms of additional capacity is not always to be expected. Table 12.1 summarizes the key stages in development and thus for therapy at the GMFCS levels during the lifespan. Specific case studies about different elements of management over the lifespan are provided in Dodd et al. (2010).

Additional areas of focus

Other important areas of CP management are physical fitness, recreational activities, maintenance of good nutrition (Sullivan 2009) and psychological well-being. There are increasing opportunities for children and adults with CP to engage in a variety of sporting and recreational activities. Although studies of the effects of these activities are less prevalent, disabled people are increasingly able to join in with leisure and sporting activities and to engage in competitive sports internationally. Some studies have shown that this can have a benefit at impairment and activity levels, but less is known about their effects on participation and quality of life.

Nutrition can be a huge challenge for some children. This is especially true for many children in GMFCS levels IV and V. The increasingly common use of feeding via gastrostomy (not necessarily to be viewed as a long-term solution), supplements and attention to diet have all helped to reduce the stress of mealtimes, so that what should be an enjoyable but often challenging activity can become less stressful for all, and safer for the person with CP.

More attention has been given to quality of life issues in recent years (discussed in Chapter 13), and there are now increasing numbers of studies about this, although many seem to focus more on the parent than the child (Raina et al. 2005; Guyard et al. 2011). Less is known about the psychological well-being of people with CP, especially children, and their families and friends. It is not known what value psychological and personal counselling (so-called 'talking therapies') has for children and adults with CP, although both are very popular approaches to therapy in many countries for the typical population and are now an integral part of National Health Service provision in the UK.

Complementary and alternative therapies

Throughout the history of medicine, there have always been both orthodox and 'alternative' approaches to the management of complex issues, and the field of CP is no exception. The so-called 'complementary and alternative medicines' (CAM) in CP involve ideas and beliefs that range from those that make some biomedical sense to those that are frankly rather fanciful when considered in the light of the modern understanding of biology in general and CP in particular.

A brief discussion of the ideas behind the proposed use of hyperbaric oxygen therapy (HBOT) for CP illustrates these points. In this approach to treating CP, the basic belief is that brain damage happens because of a lack of oxygen to the developing brain. (This has of course traditionally been a common 'explanation' for how CP occurred.) Proponents of HBOT also believed that there are areas of the brain around the oxygen-deprived damaged parts that are 'idling' (not working well but potentially susceptible to being stimulated). It is thought that forcing extra oxygen into the circulatory system under pressure ('hyperbaria') will have the effect of increasing the body's overall concentration of oxygen, thereby promoting brain function by awakening these idling areas of brain tissue. However, the 'evidence' of the effectiveness of HBOT in CP is based on testimonials from families and practitioners and studies of questionable methodological rigor (*CanChild* 2001).

Contrast these notions with today's evidence on these issues. Our current understanding of the 'causes' of CP is in fact quite different from the outdated set of ideas proposed by proponents of the use of HBOT. It is now recognized that 'hypoxic–ischaemic encepha-lopathy' is rarely a cause of the brain impairments that are associated with CP (Nelson 2003). Brain imaging studies, including ultrasound observations of the developing brain in utero, have shown clearly that many children with CP have structural and functional impairments of the brain that develop embryologically long before these infants are born. In fact, it is likely that many infants who experience perinatal distress do so specifically because they have pre-existing brain impairments that predispose them to have difficulties adapting at birth.

In other words, the traditional observations about the association between perinatal problems and the later development of CP are often accurate; however, the causal pathways that we long assumed to be at work are now recognized to have been seen because we believed in them and therefore interpreted what we saw in the light of those beliefs. What we thought were 'cause–effect' relationships are in fact 'effect–cause' con-nections. Thus, modern medicine has allowed us to understand CP in a new light, and this new understanding calls into question a basic assumption about how and why HBOT should 'work'. Nor is there evidence that parts of the brain are 'idling' and can be 'awakened' with extra oxygen.

HBOT is one of the few modern 'treatments' (orthodox or heterodox) to have been stud-ied with an excellent randomized controlled trial (Collet et al. 2001; Hardy et al. 2002). The key findings were that on virtually every outcome measure used – whether assess-ing motor function, language or cognitive abilities – children receiving a regimen of 40 hour-long sham (placebo) treatments ('dives') with slightly increased pressure and room air over 8 weeks did exactly as well as the group who received an equal number of 'real' dives with higher pressures and 100% oxygen. Thus, even if one were to argue that the exposure to slightly elevated pressure was an effective treatment (and there is no evidence to support this contention), there would be nothing to support the use of the higher pressures and 100% oxygen (and considerable costs) associated with HBOT.

One of the challenges posed by the HBOT story is that much of the current mainstream treatment in CP is not grounded in evidence as sound as that provided by the HBOT clinical trial. Clearly, all of us who work in the field have a responsibility to be as evi-dence based as the HBOT saga provoked people to be.

It is important to comment that some proponents of CAM, or other therapy ideas, can be combative and even litigious when people raise analytically critical questions or ask for sound research-based evidence to support the claims that are made about the value of these new approaches. In our view, it is inappropriate for the burden of proof to be put on the critics of a new approach; rather, we believe that is incumbent upon purvey-ors of new ideas to provide the analytically critical evidence to support their assertions.

We would of course argue that all evidence needs to be scrutinized for its rigor, to be regularly reviewed and then to be revised based on credible new findings. An example concerns the evidence to support the use of muscle strengthening for children with CP, which is needed but may not necessarily be helpful to all. Muscle strengthening had been a much-neglected area of physical therapy in the later part of the last century, but in the past decade has regained its place as an important therapy intervention. However, after being strongly recommended 10 years ago, recent evidence suggests that it might not be beneficial for all people with CP; thus, we have been required to modify our initial viewpoint about it being an essential inclusion in our clinical practice (Damiano et al. 2002, 2010). The challenge, then, is to determine what works, what works best for the individual, and in what 'dose' and at what stage of development.

In summary

The therapist's toolbox (Mayston 2007) contains many items, and the number increases as new ideas, knowledge and evidence emerge. Studies are needed to show us what strategies work best and for whom, and how and why it is that they are effective. It should also be clear from the discussion in this chapter and by others that a team approach to treatment and management is essential to enable the best outcomes for each person. This chapter does not have the scope to cover details or to mention every type of therapy or adjunctive treatment available, but hopefully provides an overview of important principles for the therapy management of CP.

References

Aarts PB, Jongerius PH, Geerdink YA, Limbeek JV, Geurts AC (2010) Effectiveness of modified constraint-induced movement therapy in children with unilateral spastic cerebral palsy: a randomized controlled trial. *Neurorehabil Neural Repair* 24: 509–18.

Anttila H, Autti-Rämö I, Suoranta J, Mäkelä M, Malmivaara A (2008) Effectiveness of physical therapy interventions for children with cerebral palsy: a systematic review. *BMC Pediatr* (Biomed Central Ltd) 24 Apr; 8: 14.

Baker R, Graham K (2011) Functional decline in children undergoing selective dorsal rhizotomy after age 10. *Dev Med Child Neurol* 53: 677.

Barrett RS (2011) What are the long-term consequences of botulinum toxin injections in spastic cerebral palsy? *Dev Med Child Neurol* 53: 485

Bélanger M, Drew T, Provencher J, Rossignol S (1996) A comparison of treadmill locomotion in adult cats before and after spinal transection. *J Neurophysiol* 76: 471–91.

Blundell SW, Shepherd RB, Dean CM, Adams RD, Cahill BM (2003): Functional strength training in cerebral palsy: a pilot study of a group circuit training class for children aged 4–8 years. *Clin Rehabil* 17: 48–57.

Bottos M, Gericke C (2003) Ambulatory capacity in cerebral palsy: prognostic criteria and consequences for intervention. *Dev Med Child Neurol* 45: 786–90.

Bourke-Taylor H, O'Shea R, Gaebler-Spira D (2007) Conductive education: a functional skills program for children with cerebral palsy. *Phys Occup Ther Pediatr* 27: 45–62.

Bower E (2009) *Finnie's Handling the Young Child with Cerebral Palsy at Home.* Oxford: Butterworth Heinemann.

Boyd R, Sakzewski L, Ziviani J et al. (2010) INCITE: A randomised trial comparing constraint induced movement therapy and bimanual training for children with congenital hemiplegia. *BMC Neurol* 12: 4.

Butler C (1986) Effects of powered mobility on self-initiated behaviors of very young children with locomotor disability. *Dev Med Child Neurol* 28: 325–32.

Butler C, Darrah J (2001) Effects of neurodevelopmental treatment (NDT) for cerebral palsy: an AACPDM evidence report. *Dev Med Child Neurol* 43: 778–90.

Butler C, Okamoto GA, McKay TM (1983) Powered mobility for very young disabled children. *Dev Med Child Neurol* 25: 472–4.

CanChild (2001) Hyperbaric oxygen therapy: hot or not? Available at: http://www.canchild.ca/en/canchil-dresources/hyperbaricoxygen.asp (accessed 7 January 2011).

Carr LJ, Harrison LM, Evans AL, Stephens JA (1993) Patterns of central motor reorganisation in hemiplegic cerebral palsy. *Brain* 116: 1223–47.

Collet JP, Vanasse M, Marois P et al. (2001) Hyperbaric oxygen for children with cerebral palsy: a randomised multicentre trial. HBOT-CP Research Group. *Lancet* 24: 582–6.

Damiano DL (2006) Activity, activity, activity: rethinking our physical therapy approach to cerebral palsy. *Phys Ther* 86: 1534–40.

Damiano DL, Abel MF (1998) Functional outcomes of strength training in spastic cerebral palsy. *Arch Phys Med Rehabil* 79: 119–25.

Damiano DL, Arnold AS, Steele KM, Delp SL (2010) Can strength training predictably improve gait kinematics? A pilot study on the effects of hip and knee extensor strengthening on lower-extremity alignment in cerebral palsy. *Phys Ther* 90: 269–79.

Darrah J, Watkins B, Chen L, Bonin C; AACPDM (2004) Conductive education intervention for children with cerebral palsy: an AACPDM evidence report. *Dev Med Child Neurol* 4: 187–203.

Darrah J, Law MC, Pollock N et al. (2011) Context therapy: a new intervention approach for children with cerebral palsy. *Dev Med Child Neurol* 53: 615–20.

Delgado MR, Hirtz D, Aisen M et al. (2010) Practice parameter: pharmacologic treatment of spasticity in children and adolescents with cerebral palsy (an evidence-based review): report of the Quality Standards Subcommittee of the American Academy of Neurology and the Practice Committee of the Child Neurology Society. *Neurology* 74: 336–43.

Desloovere K, Molenaers G, De Cat J et al. (2007) Motor function following multilevel botulinum toxin type A treatment in children with cerebral palsy. *Dev Med Child Neurol* 49: 56–61.

Dodd KJ, Foley S (2007) Partial body-weight-supported treadmill training can improve walking in children with cerebral palsy: a clinical controlled trial. *Dev Med Child Neurol* 49: 101–5.

Dodd KJ, Taylor NF, Damiano DL (2002) A systematic review of the effectiveness of strength-training programs for people with cerebral palsy. *Arch Phys Med Rehabil* 83: 1157–64.

Dodd KJ, Imms C, Taylor NF (2010). Overview of Therapy. *Physical and Occupational Therapy for People with Cerebral Palsy: A Problem Based Approach to Assessment and Management.* London: Mac Keith Press, pp. 40–72.

Duncan J (2010) Occupational therapy following upper limb surgery. In: Dodd KJ, Imms C, Taylor NF, editors. *Physical and Occupational Therapy for People with Cerebral Palsy: A Problem Based Approach to Assessment and Management.* London: Mac Keith Press, pp. 177–90.

Eliasson AC, Krumlinde-Sundholm L, Shaw K, Wang C (2005) Effects of constraint induced movement therapy in young children with hemiplegic cerebral palsy: an adapted model. *Dev Med Child Neurol* 47: 266–75.

Eliasson AC, Krumlinde Sundholm L, Rösblad B et al. (2006) The Manual Ability Classification System (MACS) for children with cerebral palsy: scale development and evidence of validity and reliability. *Dev Med Child Neurol* 48: 549–54.

Eyre JA, Smith M, Dabydeen L et al. (2007) Is hemiplegic cerebral palsy equivalent to amblyopia of the corticospinal system? *Ann Neurol* 62: 493–503.

Faigenbaum A (1999). Youth strength training: benefits, concerns and program design considerations. *Am J Med Sports* 1: 243–54.

Gericke T (2006) Postural management for children with cerebral palsy: consensus statement. *Dev Med Child Neurol* 48: 244.

Gordon AM, Chinnan A, Gill S, Petra E, Hung YC, Charles J (2008) Both constraint induced movement therapy and bimanual training lead to improved upper extremity function in children with hemiplegia. *Dev Med Child Neurol* 50: 957–8.

Graham HK, Selber P (2003) Musculoskeletal aspects of cerebral palsy. *J Bone Joint Surg* 85: 157–66.

Graham HK, Harvey A, Rodda J, Nattrass GR, Pirpiris M (2004) The Functional Mobility Scale (FMS). *J Pediatr Orthop* 24: 514–20.

Grunt S, Becher JG, Vermeulen RJ (2011) Long-term outcome and adverse effects of selective dorsal rhizotomy in children with cerebral palsy: a systematic review. *Dev Med Child Neurol* 53: 490–8.

Guyard A, Fauconnier J, Mermet MA, Cans C (2011) Impact on parents of cerebral palsy in children: a literature review. *Arch Pediatr* 18: 204–14.

Hardy P, Collet JP, Goldberg J et al. (2002) Neuropsychological effects of hyperbaric oxygen therapy in cerebral palsy. *Dev Med Child Neurol* 44: 436–46.

Harvey A, Graham HK, Morris E, Baker R, Wolfe R (2007) The Functional Mobility Scale: Ability to detect change following single event multi-level surgery. *Dev Med Child Neurol* 49: 603–7.

Harvey A (2010) Physiotherapy following single-event mulitilevel surgery (SEMLS). In: Dodd KJ, Imms C, Taylor NF, editors. *Physical and Occupational Therapy for People with Cerebral Palsy: A Problem Based Approach to Assessment and Management.* London: Mac Keith Press, pp. 159–76.

Hidecker MJC, Paneth N, Rosenbaum PL et al. (2011) Developing and validating the Communication Function Classification System (CFCS) for individuals with cerebral palsy. *Dev Med Child Neurol* 53: 704–10.

Horstman H, Bleck E (2007) *Orthopaedic Management in Cerebral Palsy*, 2nd edn. London: Mac Keith Press.

Ketelaar A, Vermeer A, Thart H, Van Petegem-van Beek E, Helders PJM (2001) Effects of a functional therapy program on motor abilities of children with cerebral palsy. *Phys Ther* 81: 1534–45.

Liao H, Liu Y, Liu W, Lin Y (2007) Effectiveness of loaded sit-to-stand resistance exercise for children with mild spastic diplegia: a randomized clinical trial. *Arch Phys Med Rehabil* 88: 25–31.

Liepert J, Bauder H, Wolfgang HR, Miltner WH, Taub E, Weiller C (2000) Treatment induced cortical reorganisation after stroke in humans. *Stroke* 31: 1210–16.

Mayston MJ (2004) Physiotherapy management in cerebral palsy: an update on treatment approaches. In: Scrutton D, Damiano D, Mayston M, editors. *Management of the Motor Disorders of CP*, 2nd edn. London: Mac Keith Press.

Mayston MJ (2007) Motor control in paediatric neurology. In Pountney T, editor. *Physiotherapy for Children.* Edinburgh: Butterworth Heinemann Elsevier, pp. 61–72.

Mayston MJ (2008) Bobath@50: midlife crisis – what of the future? Editorial. *Physiother Res Int* 13: 131–6.

Morris C, Dias LC (2007) *Paediatric Orthotics.* London: Mac Keith Press.

Morris C, Condie D (2009) *Recent Developments in Healthcare for Cerebral Palsy: Implications and Opportunities for Orthotics.* Copenhagen: International Society for Prosthetics and Orthotics. Available at: www.ispoweb. org.

Morris C, Condie D, Fisk J (2009) ISPO Cerebral Palsy Consensus Conference Report (available free at www. ispoweb.org). *Prosthet Orthot Int* 33: 401–2.

Morton RE, Gray N, Vloeberghs M (2011) Controlled study of the effects of continuous intrathecal baclofen infusion in non-ambulant children with cerebral palsy. *Dev Med Child Neurol* 53: 736–41.

Mutlu A, Krosschell K, Spira DG (2009) Treadmill training with partial body-weight support in children with cerebral palsy: a systematic review. *Dev Med Child Neurol* 51: 268–75.

Naumann M, Albanese A, Heinen F, Molenaers G, Relja M (2006) Safety and efficacy of botulinum toxin type A following long-term use. *Eur J Neurol* 13 (Suppl. 4): 35–40.

Naylor C, Bower E (2005) Modified constraint-induced movement therapy for young children with hemiplegic cerebral palsy: a pilot study. *Dev Med Child Neurol* 47: 365–9.

Nelson KB (2003) Can we prevent cerebral palsy? *N Engl J Med* 349: 1765.

Nudo RJ, Wise BM, SiFuentes F, Milliken GW (1996) Neural substrates for the effects of rehabilitative training on motor recovery after ischaemic infarct. *Science* 272: 1791–4.

Oldman P, Oberg B (2005) Effectiveness of intensive training for children with cerebral palsy – a comparison between child and youth rehabilitation and conductive education. *J Rehabil Med* 37: 263–70.

Palisano RJ, Rosenbaum PL, Walter S, Russell D, Wood E, Galuppi B (1997) Development and reliability of a system to classify gross motor function in children with cerebral palsy. *Dev Med Child Neurol* 39: 214–23.

Palisano RJ, Rosenbaum P, Bartlett D, Livingston MH (2008) Content validity of the expanded and revised Gross Motor Function Classification System. *Dev Med Child Neurol* 50: 744.

Palisano RJ, Hanna SE, Rosenbaum PL, Tieman B (2010) Probability of walking, wheeled mobility, and assisted mobility in children and adolescents with cerebral palsy. *Dev Med Child Neurol* 52: 66–71.

Pin T, Dyke P, Chan M (2006) The effectiveness of passive stretching in children with cerebral palsy. *Dev Med Child Neurol* 48: 855–62.

Raina P, O'Donnell M, Rosenbaum P et al. (2005) The health and well-being of caregivers of children with cerebral palsy. *Pediatrics* 115: e626–36.

Rosenbaum P (2003) Controversial treatment of spasticity: exploring alternative therapies for motor function in children with cerebral palsy. Review. *J Child Neurol* 18 (Suppl. 1): S89–94.

Rosenbaum PL, Gorter JW (2011) The 'F-words' in childhood disability: I swear this is how we should think! *Child Care Health Dev* doi:10.1111/j.1365-2214.2011.01338.x.

Rosenbaum PL, Walter SD, Hanna SE et al. (2002) Prognosis for gross motor function in cerebral palsy: Creation of motor development curves. *JAMA* 288: 1357–63.

Rosenbaum PL, Paneth N, Leviton A, Goldstein M, Bax M (2007) A report: the definition and classification of cerebral palsy April 2006. *Dev Med Child Neurol* 49 (Suppl. 109) : 8–14.

Russell DJ, Rosenbaum PL, Cadman DT, Gowland C, Hardy S, Jarvis S (1989) The gross motor function measure: a means to evaluate the effects of physical therapy. *Dev Med Child Neurol* 31: 341–52.

Salimi I, Friel KM, Martin JH (2008) Pyramidal tract stimulation restores normal corticospinal tract connections and visuomotor skill after early postnatal motor cortex activity blockade. *J Neurosci* 28: 7426–34.

Schindl, MR, Forstner C, Kern H, Hesse S (2000) Treadmill training with partial bodyweight support in nonambulatory patients with cerebral palsy. *Arch Phys Med Rehabil* 81: 301–6.

Scholtes VA, Becher JG, Comuth A, Dekkers H, Van Dijk L, Dallmeijer AJ (2010) Effectiveness of functional progressive resistance exercise strength training on muscle strength and mobility in children with cerebral palsy: a randomized controlled trial. *Dev Med Child Neurol* 52: e107–13.

Smyth MD, Peacock WJ (2000) The surgical treatment of spasticity. *Muscle Nerve* 23: 153–63.

Sullivan PB (2009) *Feeding and Nutrition in Children with Neurodevelopmental Disability*. London: Mac Keith Press.

Tardieu C, Lespargot A, Tabary C, Bret MD (1988) For how long must the soleus muscle be stretched each day to prevent contracture? *Dev Med Child Neurol* 30: 3–10.

Taub E, Ramey SL, DeLuca S, Echols K (2004) Efficacy of constraint induced movement therapy for children with cerebral palsy with asymmetric motor impairment. *Pediatrics* 113: 305–12.

Taylor NF, Dodd KJ, Larkin H (2004) Adults with cerebral palsy benefit from participating in a strength training programme at a community gymnasium. *Disabil Rehabil* 26: 1128–34.

Tedroff K, Löwing K, Jacobson DN, Aström E (2011) Does loss of spasticity matter? A 10-year follow-up after selective dorsal rhizotomy in cerebral palsy. *Dev Med Child Neurol* 53: 724–9.

Tefft D, Guerette P, Furumasu J (2011) The impact of early powered mobility on parental stress, negative emotions, and family social interactions. *Phys Occup Ther Pediatr* 31: 4–15.

Tuersley-Dixon L, Frederickson N (2010) Conductive education: appraising the evidence. *Educ Psychol Pract* 26: 353–73.

Willoughby KL, Dodd KJ, Shields N (2009) A systematic review of the effectiveness of treadmill training for children with cerebral palsy. *Disabil Rehabil* 31: 1971–9.

Willoughby KL, Dodd KJ, Shields N, Foley S (2010) Efficacy of partial body weight-supported treadmill training compared with overground walking practice for children with cerebral palsy: a randomized controlled trial. *Arch Phys Med Rehabil* 91: 333–9.

Wolf SL, Winstein CJ, Miller JP et al. (2008) Retention of upper limb function in stroke survivors who have received constraint-induced movement therapy: the EXCITE randomised trial. *Lancet Neurol* 7: 33–40.

World Confederation for Physical Therapy (2011) Physiotherapy. Essential to your health, mobility and independence. Available at: http://www.wcpt.org/sites/wcpt.org/files/files/Publicity_materials-CPA-Physiotherapy_essential_to_your_health.pdf (accessed 12 March 2011).

World Federation of Occupational Therapists (2011). What is occupational therapy? Available at: http://www.wfot.org/AboutUs/AboutOccupationalTherapy/WhatisOccupationalTherapy.aspx (accessed 12 March 2011).

Part 4

Outcomes in childhood and beyond

Chapter 13

Outcomes

Overview

The issues of 'outcome' in people with cerebral palsy (CP) are multilayered. In the first part of this chapter we address what people might mean by 'outcomes'. We indicate that in order to be helpful to people, before we respond we need to clarify their questions. Doing so makes it more likely that we will answer the specific question we are being asked by a parent, a colleague or a policy-maker. The answers we provide depend in part on the tools used to assess those outcomes, who is asking, what exactly they are asking, what their frames of reference are, how 'outcomes' are being defined and the time course under consideration. The purpose of identifying these factors is simply to remind people that, as always, the answers depend on the precision of the questions. In the second part of the chapter we discuss quality of life (QoL) and suggested ways to determine people's outcome goals.

What outcomes, as judged by whom?

Among the most common questions concerning people with CP is 'How do these children "do" over time?' This is a perfectly reasonable concern, but as readers will appreciate it is also a complex question to answer simply because there are many dimensions of the question to be considered. Before addressing specific issues directly, it is important to outline the reasons why this apparently straightforward question must be considered carefully in order for any responses to make sense. This includes understanding the context of the question. To get at the context requires a recognition that different players in the CP 'story' have different expectations about a variety of outcomes. A brief overview of these larger considerations is in order, with some examples to illustrate what we have in mind.

In 1991, Goldberg wrote an important article about the need for professionals to recognize that we must consider and address three kinds of outcomes: technical, functional health and patient satisfaction. Technical outcomes refer to the 'objective' observations of change after an intervention. These might be measured radiologically (e.g. spinal alignment after instrumentation) or with simple instruments (e.g. joint range of motion assessed with a goniometer) or clinically (e.g. changes in spasticity). In all of these examples it is the practitioner to whom the outcome is of interest. And of course it is essential that as clinicians we evaluate whether we achieve the 'outcomes' of the treatments we have recommended – both in the individual case and in the population to whom such interventions are prescribed. Only through evidence accumulated systematically, validly and reliably can we have some confidence that these interventions can/will produce the desired outcomes in the specific situation and do more good than harm.

Goldberg's second category of outcomes refers to those that affect what he referred to as 'functional health'. For many people, including parents and children with CP, these might be colloquially called the 'so what?' outcomes. These address the question of whether technical outcomes made a difference to the functional well-being of the people who received them. In International Classification of Functioning, Disability and Health (ICF) (World Health Organization 2001) terms (see Chapter 7), these outcomes might be categorized as affecting 'activity' or 'participation' – aspects of people's lives that are generally likely to be of more interest to them than the technical changes described above. Note how the change of perspective on the success and value of any specific outcome can change the whole discussion of 'outcomes'.

Of course, if an intervention is directed at improving pain, which might be categorized within the 'body structure and function' level of the ICF, most people would consider any success of an intervention directed at this 'technical' outcome to be tremendously important. Note, however, that such an outcome would also have been a patient-identified goal, would probably have spill-over effects on people's activity and participation and may in fact provide at least some of the evidence of success of the intervention. The same would not automatically be the case with a change in alignment of a limb after other technical interventions, as these do not necessarily translate to improved activity or participation (Wright et al. 2007).

The third category of outcomes described by Goldberg are those that concern patient satisfaction, and here, as outlined in Chapter 8, we would include parent and family satisfaction. This kind of outcome, reported by the person making the evaluation, presumably includes a summative judgement of the technical and functional outcomes that they or their child have experienced. However, as proposed elsewhere, we believe that there can be outcomes of the processes of service delivery that do not depend solely on the technical and functional outcomes but stand as separate important markers that we believe can and should be targets of the services and interventions we provide.

Measuring outcomes: what kinds of tools do we need?

The nature of the outcome of interest should determine what kind of measures we need to use to get the best (truest, most valid) answers. A very brief introduction to measures is in order because, as we will show, one needs the right 'tools' for the job, whatever that job might be. Needless to say, the methods used to accumulate information about outcomes will also be extremely important when it comes to assessing the credibility of the findings.

In reality, measures are simply tools used to address a specific task. Think of a tape measure used to assess a child's head circumference, a scale to assess a person's weight or a cuff to measure blood pressure. Whether we are talking about a technically simple tool like a tape measure to assess size or a more sophisticated machine like a magnetic resonance scanner to explore the inner structure and workings of the body, each instrument needs to be able to evaluate what it measures reliably (i.e. consistently). Only under these circumstances can we have confidence that a specific reading is representative of the observations made with that tool. In addition, each instrument must provide a valid (i.e. 'true') indication of the characteristic being measured or assessed.

It is also important to specify the purpose for which a measure is needed so that the right tools are selected for the job (Rosenbaum 1998). To assess whether something is present or absent, or to judge the degree to which it is present, one needs measures that have been shown to discriminate the characteristic of interest. To predict the future status of a person, one needs measures (and research designs) that are known to have the capacity to provide such information. To assess change one must use evaluative methods that are known to be capable of measuring meaningful change over time when such a change has indeed happened.

In order to consider the kinds of questions one might ask and the tools needed to answer each of these questions, we will illustrate what we mean by providing examples that concern gross motor function.

Suppose a young child presents to a community clinic because of concerns about motor 'delay'. People might use a screening instrument to 'discriminate' whether the child's function is within the expected range for typical development (they 'pass' the screening test) or outside that range (they 'fail' and screen 'positive' and need further assessment). For this kind of measurement exercise we need tools that are 'norm referenced'. These are measures that have been appropriately developed with populations that are similar to that from which the child in the clinic comes. Screening tests are an example of norm-referenced discriminative tools that allow us to see whether someone performs 'well enough' to pass the screening assessment. If the child 'fails' the screening test, we then need to look at them carefully to see whether they do indeed have a problem and whether we can detect an explanation for their difficulties.

When a child presents with definite CP, parents may ask 'How bad is it?' This questions requires another kind of measure or classification tool, one that again can discriminate. In this case our interest is in using a condition-specific instrument to fit the child into one of a varying number of levels of function that are known to be importantly distinct and are also meaningful to parents. These are provided by instruments such as the Gross Motor Function Classification System (GMFCS) (Palisano et al. 1997, 2008) (see Appendix I). The five GMFCS levels discriminate what we know to be important and relatively stable (Palisano et al. 2006) variations in gross motor function, and this information is known to be useful to parents when they are ready to ask.

Parents may also want to know 'Will our child walk?' This is clearly a question of prediction of future status, and requires two elements. The first is a way of describing current function, such as is done with the GMFCS, so that there is a common language to describe the starting points from which the prediction is being made. The second and in many ways more important component is evidence from prospective (forward-looking) studies that have systematically tracked the 'outcome' of interest (in this case, gross motor mobility). If one has reliable and valid information about later function and can relate that outcome to earlier 'markers' of function, a prediction can be made. Findings from the Ontario Motor Growth Study (Rosenbaum et al. 2002) have indicted clearly that we can answer parents' questions about future mobility with a high degree of accuracy after the age of 2 years (Wood and Rosenbaum 2000), using the GMFCS as the indicator (measure) with which to predict (Appendix V).

A motor measurement question from clinicians and researchers usually concerns what tools to use to assess changes in function over time or in response to an intervention. Here one needs measures that have been validated as change-detecting tools. As we wrote many years ago (Rosenbaum et al. 1990), when people are unaware of the functions of tools they can easily misapply what seem like good measures and be disappointed by the results. In the early days of studying CP, many of the tools available to us had been developed using children who did not necessarily have CP. They were also almost always norm-referenced measures which were useful to discriminate levels of function but often expressly designed not to assess change.

Think, for example, of IQ tests, where the scoring involves computing a 'raw' score of current performance and dividing that value by the child's age to derive the 'quotient'. Over time a typical child acquires huge increases in knowledge and skills, but their IQ rarely changes very much. The reason is that the denominator keeps changing (i.e. increasing) because the child is older each time they are assessed. Using traditional IQ tests to assess changes in knowledge and skills will clearly lead one to conclude that the child is no better off as they grow, when the opposite is clearly the case.

To assess motor function in children with CP, one needs to use purpose-designed evaluative measures like the Gross Motor Function Measure (Russell et al. 2002) and the Pediatric Evaluation of Disability Inventory (Haley et al. 1992). Both measures were developed and validated specifically for their capacity to detect change when change was judged to have happened, and to provide consistent scores over time in situations where function was stable.

To return to the theme of this aspect of the 'outcomes' story, our ability to answer questions about outcomes will depend powerfully on whether we have the right tools for the job for that evaluation and whether the studies on which we base our answers were designed appropriately to provide such an answer. These broad 'critical appraisal' issues were reviewed in Chapter 6.

The time course of outcomes

We ask about how people with CP do 'over time'. This reflects the importance of being clear about the time course we have in mind in trying to answer the question. As described above, even this question might mean different things to different questioners. Parents often have different outcomes in mind than professionals and almost certainly are thinking about a different time course.

Realistically, most of what we know about the outcomes of most health conditions has been gleaned from observations over relatively short time intervals. Research on specific interventions usually explores the outcomes after several months, or perhaps after as long as a couple of years, whereas the questioner (for example a programme manager or policy-maker) might have a longer period in mind. Thus, with the exception of crude outcome markers like survival, we often simply lack information about outcomes over the course of many years.

There are many reasons for this dilemma. For one thing, it can be very difficult to make long-term formal observations of the type systematically undertaken in research studies. One of the practical reasons is that specific research studies are usually funded for 2 or 3 or, occasionally, 5 years, and even then the actual period of observation of the outcomes of interest is usually briefer than that. Thus, the longer-term technical outcomes may be poorly known.

Another reality is that when trying to attribute specific outcomes to specific interventions, we need to recognize that many other factors are also potentially influencing that outcome concurrently. These include children's natural development, additional interventions they may be receiving, their health status, their own preferences for the activities they choose to pursue or avoid and the amount of effort they put into that activity.

It is hopefully obvious that in response to the question 'How do these children do over time?' we need to know who is asking the question and clarify the meaning behind the question as posed. This applies whether the questioner is a parent, a professional, a manager, a policy analyst making resource decisions or a member of the public.

Quality of life

A relatively modern focus on outcomes concerns the QoL of people with virtually any health challenge. It is important to provide a brief overview of the QoL theme, because even as we enter the second decade of the twenty-first century these ideas are still being developed, clarified, debated and measured in a host of ways that are, at times, in conflict with each other. The ideas that follow reflect the authors' personal views (perhaps even biases), but might hopefully still be helpful to others by discussing some of the issues involved.

The notion of QoL has been adopted and is increasingly being promoted across the community. It is hard to find a daily newspaper in which the phrase 'quality of life' is not used regularly. Politicians argue that their policies improve the 'quality of life' of voters. Advertisers assure us that their products and services will enhance our 'quality of life'. In the health field, an interest in people's 'quality of life' has reached a crescendo of attention in the past decade or more, to the point at which virtually everyone wants to measure this 'outcome' either as a description of the well-being of people with a condition or as an outcome of an intervention.

It is important to distinguish two broad concepts: what people refer to as 'health-related quality of life' (HRQOL) – the way in which a condition (almost always a chronic condition) affects people's well-being – and what we like to refer to as people's 'existential' QoL, meaning their personal assessment and valuation of their life condition. The former approach is consistent with the ideas inherent in the ICF (see Chapter 7). That approach has evolved because of a recognition that we need to be aware of the impact of a condition on a person's life and function, and not simply on their biomedical status. These issues have been discussed by Livingston et al. (2007) and Rosenbaum (2007); the argument about the differences in these perspectives is illustrated with data from Rosenbaum et al. (2007).

This expanded interest in function and well-being represents, for us, an important widening of the scope of outcomes that we believe we should be considering as we work with people with chronic conditions. Within these outcomes, one should distinguish the generic (widely applicable) 'health status' measures that describe people's function across a range of dimensions (an example in the adult field is the SF-36; Ware and Sherbourne 1992) and what are often referred to as multi-attribute utility measures, which have been developed by economists specifically to take account of the values ('utilities') that people place on these health states (an example is the Health Utilities Index; Feeny et al. 1996). The former measures are descriptive and allow us to compare the health status of people with different conditions. The latter measures make it possible in addition to ascribe a community-derived utility or value (usually ranging from 0.0 [death] to 1.0 [perfect health]) to each specific combination of functional states of the people being measured. These utilities can then be compared across disorders, treatments, communities, etc.

Note, however, that while these HRQOL measures have usually been termed measures of QoL, we prefer to think of them as measures of functional status. For one thing, the 'quality' or values ascribed to these health states in the utility measures are not those of the people who have the conditions, but are derived from community citizens at large. It has been recognized (Albrecht and Devlieger 1999) that, apparently paradoxically, people with significant observable functional limitations can self-assess their QoL to be very good. These research findings point to the distinction between what outsiders consider the (reduced) value of a health state to be (perhaps how they imagine they might feel in that health state) and the perspectives and judgements of the people who live with those health states and apparently view their world through an entirely different lens.

Our own work with adolescents with CP allowed us to contrast objectively measured HRQOL, and the utilities associated with those observations, and the self-assessed QoL of these same young people. There were very striking differences between the utility findings, many of which varied significantly by severity of motor limitations, and the results obtained with a measure that asked young people about their lives with respect to 'being, belonging, becoming' (which did not vary systematically by motor impairment). In other words, the young people's perceptions of their lives were apparently not conditioned by what others might judge to be poorer functional status (Rosenbaum et al. 2007). The head-to-head relationship between these two sets of observations was very weak, indicating that they are in fact measuring quite different dimensions (outcomes) of people's lives.

Determining outcomes

There is an increasing interest in looking at patient-reported outcomes (e.g. the US Food and Drug Administration [http://www.fda.gov/AboutFDA/PartnershipsCollaborations/ PublicPrivatePartnershipProgram/ucm231129.htm; accessed 20 March 2012] and the INVOLVE programme [http://www.invo.org.uk/] in the UK). This move reflects an awareness in the field of health services that professionals need to know what patient goals are in treatment and assess these to the best of our ability. We have made reference throughout the book to the study by Ketelaar and colleagues (2001) that illustrated the importance of engaging with both families and children to identify their goals in treatment, to tailor interventions appropriately and to assess the achievement of those goals.

An assessment tool that was purpose built and is widely used to achieve the identification of patient goals is the Canadian Occupational Performance Measure (COPM) (Law et al. 1998). The COPM is based on a model of occupational 'performance' that includes a person's identification of their goals for self-care, productivity and leisure (McColl et al. 2005). Using prompts from the interviewer, the respondent identifies issues in an area of occupational performance that they want, need or are expected to do but with which they are having difficulty, or with which they are not satisfied with 'how it's going' currently. Identified issues in occupational performance are rated in terms of importance on a scale of 1–10 (1=not important at all, 10=very important). The five 'most important issues' are then identified by the individual and rated in terms of both performance and satisfaction. After an intervention directed at addressing those goals, the respondent identifies their current valuation of these areas and makes a judgement about whether and how much the achievement of these goals has changed. There is good evidence that the COPM can be used with parents of young children (Cusick et al. 2007). Work in Canada used the COPM to identify the issues of concern to adolescents with CP (Livingston et al. 2011).

Another well-known approach to goal setting and assessment is Goal Attainment Scaling (GAS) (see Steenbeek et al. [2007] for a review of its use in paediatrics). In GAS specific goals are set, following which two levels are described that represent success beyond the goal as well as two of levels of lack of achievement (King et al. 1999). Novak et al. (2009) and Wallen et al. (2007) have both used GAS effectively in studies of children with CP. Cusick et al. (2006) undertook an exploration of both the COPM and GAS and concluded that both were effective and that the choice of outcome approach should depend on study aim and logistic and resource factors. Based on their study with preschoolers with CP, Ostensjø et al. (2008) recommended using a combination of the two measures, and commented that when this was done '. . . a dynamic and interactive process of setting and implementing goals in the context of everyday activities emerged'. McDougall and Wright (2009) presented ideas about how GAS can be used in conjunction with the child and young person version of the ICF (ICF-CY) to provide an approach to outcome identification that engages parents (i.e. is family centred) and is standardized.

Finally, it is worth identifying an example of the kind of evidence-based information that we would like to have about the long-term outcomes of people with CP across many areas of function. As reported earlier in this chapter, the Ontario Motor Growth study (Rosenbaum et al. 2002) assessed the gross motor function of a randomly selected community-based population of several hundred children and young people with CP over a 4-year period. Using purpose-designed measures it was possible to chart distinct patterns of motor function for each level of the GMFCS. This prospective longitudinal study was followed by a second phase of assessment of over 200 of these young people during their adolescent years (Hanna et al. 2009). These added perspectives helped to identify that there appear to be declines in measured motor function in some subgroups of the population. This kind of information is important when counselling families and young people with CP. It also challenges professionals to look carefully at those groups in which decline is a risk, to understand the mechanisms behind these changes and to explore interventions that might prevent or retard these declines.

With the availability of validated classification systems that describe levels of function in manual abilities (Eliasson et al. 2006) and communication (Hidecker et al. 2011), there are now opportunities to undertake similar studies on the long-term functional outcomes of people with CP. As noted elsewhere, it is only with systematic prospective longitudinal research that looks serially at the functional performance of the same people over many years that we will confidently be able to know what these 'outcomes' really look like. Other aspects of these issues are addressed in Chapter 12.

References

Albrecht GL, Devlieger PJ (1999) The disability paradox: high quality of life against all odds. *Soc Sci Med* 48: 977–88.

Cusick A, McIntyre S, Novak I, Lannin N, Lowe KA (2006) Comparison of goal attainment scaling and the Canadian Occupational Performance Measure for paediatric rehabilitation research. *Pediatr Rehabil* 9: 149–57.

Cusick A, Lannin NA, Lowe K (2007) Adapting the Canadian Occupational Performance Measure for use in a paediatric clinical trial. *Disabil Rehabil* 29: 761–6.

Eliasson AC, Krumlinde Sundholm L, Rösblad B et al. (2006) The Manual Ability Classification System (MACS) for children with cerebral palsy: scale development and evidence of validity and reliability. *Dev Med Child Neurol* 48: 549–54.

Feeny DH, Torrance GW, Furlong WJ (1996) Health Utilities Index. In: Spilker B, editor. *Quality of Life and Pharmacoeconomics in Clinical Trials*, 2nd edn. Philadelphia: Lippincott-Raven, pp. 239–52.

Goldberg MJ (1991) Measuring outcomes in cerebral palsy. *J Pediatr Orthop* 11: 682–5.

Haley SM, Coster WJ, Ludlow LH et al. (1992) *Pediatric Evaluation of Disability Inventory: Development, Standardization, and Administration Manual*, Version 1.0. Boston: New England Medical Center.

Hanna SE, Rosenbaum PL, Bartlett DJ et al. (2009) Stability and decline in gross motor function among children and youth with cerebral palsy aged 2 to 21 years. *Dev Med Child Neurol* 51: 295–302.

Hidecker MJC, Paneth N, Rosenbaum PL et al. (2011) Developing and validating the Communication Function Classification System (CFCS) for individuals with cerebral palsy. *Dev Med Child Neurol* 53: 704–10.

Ketelaar M, Vermeer A, Hart H et al. (2001) Effects of a functional therapy program on motor abilities of children with CP. *Phys Ther* 81: 1534–45.

King GA, McDougall J, Palisano RJ, Gritzan J, Tucker MA (1999) Goal attainment scaling: Its use in evaluating pediatric therapy programs. *Phys Occup Ther Pediatr* 19: 31–52.

Law M, Baptiste S, McColl M, Carswell A, Polatajko H, Pollock N (1998) *Canadian Occupational Performance Measure (COPM) Manual*, 3rd edn. Ottawa, ON: CAOT Publications ACE.

Livingston M, Rosenbaum PL, Russell D, Palisano RJ (2007) Quality of life among adolescents with cerebral palsy: descriptive and measurement issues. *Dev Med Child Neurol* 49: 225–31.

Livingston MH, Stewart D, Rosenbaum PL, Russell DJ (2011) Exploring issues of participation among adolescents with cerebral palsy: what's important to them? *Phys Occup Ther Pediatr* 31: 275–87.

McColl MA, Law M, Baptiste S, Pollock N, Carswell A, Polatajko HJ (2005) Targeted applications of the Canadian Occupational Performance Measure. *Can J Occup Ther* 72: 298–300.

McDougall J, Wright V (2009) The ICF-CY and Goal Attainment Scaling: benefits of their combined use for pediatric practice. *Disabil Rehabil* 31(16): 1362–72.

Novak I, Cusik A, Lannin N (2009) Occupational therapy home programs for cerebral palsy: a double blind, randomized controlled trial. *Pediatrics* 124: e606–14.

Ostensjø S, Oien I, Fallang B (2008) Goal-oriented rehabilitation of preschoolers with cerebral palsy – a multi-case study of combined use of the Canadian Occupational Performance Measure (COPM) and the Goal Attainment Scaling (GAS). *Dev Neurorehabil* 11: 252–9.

Palisano R, Rosenbaum P, Walter S, Russell D, Wood E, Galuppi B (1997) Development and reliability of a system to classify gross motor function in children with cerebral palsy. *Dev Med Child Neurol* 39: 214–23.

Palisano R, Cameron D, Rosenbaum PL, Walter SD, Russell D (2006) Stability of the Gross Motor Function Classification System. *Dev Med Child Neurol* 48: 424–8.

Palisano RJ, Rosenbaum P, Bartlett D, Livingston MH (2008) Content validity of the Expanded and Revised Gross Motor Function Classification System. *Dev Med Child Neurol* 50: 744.

Rosenbaum PL (1998) Screening tests and standardized assessments used to identify and characterize developmental delays. *Semin Pediatr Neurol* 5: 1–7.

Rosenbaum P (2007) Children's quality of life: separating the person from the disorder. *Arch Dis Child* 92: 100–1.

Rosenbaum P, Cadman D, Russell D, Gowland C, Hardy S, Jarvis S (1990) Issues in measuring change in motor function in children with cerebral palsy. A special communication. *Phys Ther* 70: 125–31.

Rosenbaum PL, Walter SD, Hanna SE et al. (2002) Prognosis for Gross Motor Function in Cerebral Palsy: creation of motor development curves. *JAMA* 288: 1357–63.

Rosenbaum PL, Livingston MH, Palisano RJ, Galuppi BE, Russell DJ (2007) Quality of life and health-related quality of life of adolescents with cerebral palsy. *Dev Med Child Neurol* 49: 516–21.

Russell D, Rosenbaum PL, Avery L, Lane M (2002) *The Gross Motor Function Measure. GMFM-66 and GMFM-88 (Users' Manual)*. Clinics in Developmental Medicine No. 159. London: Mac Keith Press.

Steenbeek D, Ketelaar M, Galama K, Gorter JW (2007) Goal attainment scaling in paediatric rehabilitation: a critical review of the literature. *Dev Med Child Neurol* 49: 550–6.

Wallen M, O'Flaherty SJ, Waugh MC (2007) Functional outcomes of intramuscular botulinum toxin type and occupational therapy in the upper limbs of children with cerebral palsy: A randomized controlled trial. *Arch Phys Med Rehabil* 88: 1–10.

Ware JE Jr, Sherbourne CD (1992) The MOS 36-item short-form health survey (SF-36). I. Conceptual framework and item selection. *Med Care* 30: 473–83.

Wood E, Rosenbaum P (2000) The Gross Motor Function Classification System for cerebral palsy: a study of reliability and stability over time. *Dev Med Child Neurol* 42: 292–6.

World Health Organization (2001) International Classification of Functioning, Disability and Health. Geneva: World Health Organization.

Wright FV, Rosenbaum PL, Fehlings D (2007) How do changes in impairment, activity, and participation relate to each other? Study of children with cerebral palsy (CP) who have received lower extremity botulinum toxin type-A (Bt-A) injections. *Dev Med Child Neurol* 50: 283–9.

Chapter 14

Transition to adulthood

Overview

Cerebral palsy (CP) is referred to as a 'children's disease' in so far as it becomes clinically evident very early in life. Most diagnostic, therapy, educational and other services for people with CP are concentrated on the needs of developing children and their families, as outlined in several chapters of this book. We know, however, that children with CP become adults with CP, and issues concerning adults with CP are discussed in the final chapter of this book.

Transition to adulthood is recognized to be a challenging developmental phase for most young people. For those with lives complicated by chronic conditions, and certainly for those with neurodevelopmental disabilities such as CP, this transition can be particularly challenging. In this chapter we offer perspectives on contextual aspects of this phase of development, considering elements of the social, educational and service dimensions of the lives of young people with CP. We then review specific issues concerning the health and function of young people emerging into adulthood and identify areas for further development at both the service and research levels.

Transition: the social context

Over the past decade or more, there has been an increasing recognition of the challenges faced by disabled young people as they make the transition in later adolescence from the world of child-orientated services to the 'adult' world (Binks et al. 2007; Rosenbaum and Stewart 2007; Roebroeck et al. 2009). It is important that these contextual considerations be identified so that planning for this developmental phase of life can be undertaken early and effectively. The opening section of this chapter discusses these issues and points to opportunities to help young people (and their families) make these transitions as smoothly as possible.

It has been noted elsewhere (see Chapter 10) that we think of parenting as a dance led by the children. That is to say, typically developing children and young people are constantly taking the initiative to try things (leading the dance). Parents can use each new 'adventure' as an opportunity to teach, offer advice and provide corrective feedback. This is how young people develop a sense of self – through experiences and the learning associated with those experiences. This reality is an essential component of the process of all development.

When young people grow up with differences and disabilities during their developing years, it may not be as easy for them to take charge of their lives, or for their parents to 'allow' them to make decisions for themselves. If this is the case then transition to adulthood may be especially challenging for everyone, parents and young people alike.

As child health professionals who work with infants and children with disabilities like CP and other chronic conditions, our connections with the children actually begin as relationships with fellow adults (the parents). The child may be the 'patient', but it is the parents who express the worries and with whom we plan the course of action. They are the people who bring the children to us, who ask the questions, whose predicaments we address – in fact, they are the people with whom we work.

It can be challenging to change that social dynamic as the children become old enough to speak for themselves. But this shift of focus is an essential development, so that we can begin to understand how young people view their lives and what their issues are. By the adolescent years, and even in the childhood years, health professionals should begin to work directly with young people with CP and not see their lives only through their parents' eyes. That changing dynamic can set a tone for the family as well, illustrating to them that their children usually have their own perspectives and needs, to which we must pay attention. When we start this process of respecting the children's voices as well as those of their parents, we are then in a position, in the adolescent years, to set the stage for transition planning with the young person as well as their family.

The processes of developing one's own identity begin in childhood and are especially important in adolescence as young people define their interests and start to plot a course for themselves. This aspect of child development is at least as important for young people with developmental challenges such as CP, in which much of our traditional early emphasis has been on disability rather than on capability, and on 'therapies' traditionally designed to promote 'normality'. As discussed in Chapters 7 and 8, a strengths-based approach to child and family issues provides opportunities to understand, from the children and young people themselves, what their goals and interests are, and then, to the extent possible, use that information to help them achieve those goals.

Nieuwenhuijsen et al. (2009) used the Canadian Occupational Performance Measure (COPM) (Law et al. 2005) with 87 intellectually capable young people with CP. The study focused on the problems being experienced by the group. These included issues in daily life, addressing the areas of self-care (59%), productivity (52%) and leisure (37%). Problems were most prevalent in recreation and leisure (30%), preparing meals (29%), housework (14%) and dressing (14%). From the perspective of the young people themselves, issues in functional mobility, paid or unpaid work and socialization were considered as the most important (represented by the highest mean importance score). Mobility problems were associated with lower levels of gross motor functioning, and problems with self-care were associated with lower levels of manual ability.

Recent work with 203 adolescents, aged 13–20 years, with CP has also helped to identify their issues in their own words (Livingston et al. 2011). This study included young people with CP across the full range of functional and intellectual abilities. Again, using the COPM, the themes that the adolescents identified most frequently were related to active leisure (identified by 57% of participants), mobility (access and getting around as well as physical issues; 55%), school (48%) and socialization (44%). Interestingly there was no association between the total number of issues identified and sex, age, type of respondent (adolescents or parent) or level of gross motor function.

This kind of emerging evidence provides a basis for seeing these young people as more typical of adolescents than as different from them. It can be very useful in our conversations with both young people and their parents to indicate our expectations that they be ready to identify how they want the next phase of their life to unfold beyond the 'CP' elements that may have been the primary focus until that point, and perhaps have been how they have been encouraged to see themselves previously.

Transition: the educational context

In many communities children and young people with disabilities like CP were traditionally segregated into 'special' schools that emphasized differences at the expense of commonalities. In the process, and with the focus on the functional 'differences' that led to the segregation, educators and others might have underestimated the potential for these young people to achieve success in academic and social pursuits. Programmes that promote integration of children and disabled young people into mainstream education have largely supplanted these traditions, making it possible for disabled young people to have a more typical, community-based educational experience. However, one cannot help wondering whether the educational expectations of disabled young people are still limited, and therefore worry that the academic horizons of these young people will be constrained because of their disabilities or because of people's assumptions based on those disabilities. Of course, we accept that for some young people with CP it is likely that cognitive limitations will clearly restrict opportunities for higher education.

We believe that with adequate accommodations for learning challenges, accurate cognitive assessment by expert educational psychologists, and appropriate technical supports, many young people with CP and other disabilities can be helped to realize their academic potential and their career aspirations. In this mode of thinking, the educational and social challenge, as outlined in more detail in Chapter 7, is to recognize and exploit 'capacity' rather than to be constrained by a young person's apparent limitations in 'performance'.

We all recognize that anecdotal experiences provide, at best, tantalizing examples of what might be possible. Having said that, here are two interesting experiences. One of the authors currently works with a former child patient with CP (Gross Motor Function Classification System [GMFCS] level IV, using a power wheelchair), who is now an articulate young colleague in his early 30s who holds a master's degree in political science and is pursuing a PhD in rehabilitation science. We would not even have considered this scenario possible 30 years ago – this simply was not what people with CP 'did'. A second example involves a young woman, a former patient with a hemisyndrome and epilepsy, who acquired a master's degree in social work and has pursued a productive career of service and advocacy for disadvantaged citizens.

These personal experiences of young people's life trajectories simply illustrate that we need to be very careful not to judge the book by the cover, but to understand the capabilities and life goals of disabled young people and strive to support them and their families in realizing their ambitions.

Transition: the services context

It might be said that young people with developmental disabilities become 'orphans' in the adult healthcare arena. Conditions like CP may phenotypically resemble adult-onset disabilities like acquired brain injury or spinal cord injury. However, the life-course trajectories of people with CP are substantially different from those of people with adult-onset disabilities (Stewart et al. 2001). As a consequence, the service sector may not understand either the needs or the capabilities of young adults with CP. One hears stories of health professionals ascribing any health problem expressed by an adult with CP to their underlying condition, and as a result misdiagnosing, and missing, serious problems such as acute gall bladder disease.

Life after school

For those children with CP who attend mainstream schools and those who attend specialist schools, transition theoretically includes plans for further or higher education, discussion of employment prospects, planning for relevant social activities, changes in healthcare provision and planning for increased independence. Models of provision for all of these vary, and for many families they can be perceived to be limited, in both their extent and their usefulness.

In general, it is our experience that facilities are more available to those with mild degrees of disability and it is easy, therefore, to comment on the paucity of provision for those who are most severely affected. Thus, there may be little choice for families but to continue to care for a severely disabled and dependent individual in their own homes.

Transition: the clinical context

Evidence from quality of life (QoL) studies (Dickinson et al. 2007) suggests that children with CP who are in the 8–12 years age group in Europe perceive themselves in general as having a similar QoL to other children. These data are derived from the Study of Participation of Children Living in Europe (SPARCLE) study using the KIDSCREEN instrument (www.kidscreen.de).

Transitions towards adulthood are taxing for typically developing young people. The specific additional difficulties for those with CP may relate to motor functioning, capacity to undertake self-help and daily living activities, oromotor function and nutrition, planning for school leaving and further or higher education including university entrance, prospects for employment, capacity for social independence, relationships and sexuality, and health.

Gross motor function

Evidence from Hanna et al. (2009) confirms that among children and young people at GMFCS levels III–V there is, for some, a degree of clinically significant deterioration in their motor function as determined by Gross Motor Function Measure scores up to the age of 21 years. Knowing that their motor function and, for example, their degree of dependence on wheelchair transport can be predicted from much earlier in childhood, it is our view that adaptation to limitations in independent walking should precede adolescence. Individuals at levels III–V, together with their families and involved professionals, should have ensured that appropriate provisions and adaptations to these potential changes in mobility needs are in place.

However, within this grouping it is important to promote pain-free and comfortable seated and other postures. In fact, in the SPARCLE study (Dickinson et al. 2007) pain was correlated with a lower self-reported QoL in 8- to 12-year-olds. It follows that the provision of appropriate seating, wheelchairs and orthoses together, when necessary, with advice on relevant orthopaedic surgical procedures should be components of management in children entering adolescence.

Decisions on how best to maintain independent mobility for those at GMFCS levels I and II may be more difficult. Indeed, effective independence in some environments may best be provided for many by wheelchairs or other transport (including adapted motor vehicles) rather than by ambulation (Tieman et al. 2004). This is likely to be the case when significant energy levels are required for walking and when public transport facilities are limited.

Within this context there is often a tension among those with CP, their families, and physical and occupational therapists with respect to the emphases that are required to maintain assisted standing and walking on the one hand and maximizing mobility and independence on the other. When this occurs, it should be possible to resolve the issues if appropriate therapeutic aims can be identified and agreed on early in adolescence.

(It is worth reminding able-bodied readers that we too may choose to take a lift or escalator rather than walk up a few flights of stairs, even when we are perfectly capable of doing so. Thus, the use of 'technical aids' such as lifts does not automatically imply a lack of capacity or a failure of functional ability. Choice is part of everyone's daily life experience, and should not be overinterpreted as evidence of loss when choices like these are made by disabled people.)

One aspect of maintenance of motor functioning that is important is to ensure that physical fitness is prioritized. This can be achieved using appropriate exercise activities, and these should be a component of societal participation for young people with CP wherever possible within community-based programmes as opposed to 'therapies'. Examples include wheelchair sports and swimming. It is a significant component of the role of the physical therapist to devise and advise on suitable physical activity programmes for individual adolescents.

A small number of young people are exceptional with respect to their physical skills. One example is the young woman, a former patient, who took an opportunity to 'drop in' to the clinic to explain that she is now a funded professional athlete. She is a member of the national boccia team. She is at GMFCS level III and has patchy cognitive impairments, but more than compensates for this by her competitive drive and achievements.

A further relevant aspect of mobility is whether young people with CP can learn to drive a motor vehicle, usually with, but sometimes without, adaptations. We take the view that appropriate assessments should be undertaken in the early teenage years whenever this is possible. For those who can successfully drive, this ability adds impressively to their potential for independence.

Self-help and daily living activities
The degree of competence of individuals with CP with respect to undertaking daily living activities is usually apparent from quite early in childhood. This applies particularly to feeding, dressing and undressing, bathing and other aspects of self-care. The key to maximizing and maintaining these functions into adult life resides principally in advising upon and providing appropriate environmental adaptations and expectations for independence. These include appropriately adapted accessible accommodation and, within this, the provision of other relevant aids and equipment that facilitate bathing and using the toilet.

Within this context, it is our experience that if urinary and faecal continence are going to be achieved in individuals, it is exceptional for this to happen any later than 8 years of age. In practice this also seems to apply to those who have sufficiently preserved cognition for there to have been an expectation that they would become continent in the pre-adolescent years.

There is an absence of relevant studies that offer information and guidance on this aspect of maturation and self-care. The achievement of continence is likely to depend on multiple factors. These will include individual and family motivation, the provision of appropriate teaching and the availability of appropriate domestic facilities. Some specific issues such as appropriate management of constipation may also be relevant.

Clearly, however, the issue of continence is a significant factor that requires consideration when examining the prospects for independence and the pattern of care needs that will be required in adolescence and adult life.

Oromotor function and nutrition
The acquisition of intelligible speech can be promoted and maintained by appropriate interventions in childhood. Against that background there is an innate drive to communicate using speech, even when intelligibility is severely compromised. The capacity of family members to understand and respond to what is being said to them by a child with CP can be very impressive indeed.

Often the challenge is to find ways to enable young people to be comprehensible to others who do not know them as well as their families. In this respect alternative and augmented forms of communication can be essential for functioning and interaction not only within the family but also, and indeed to a greater extent, in activities away from the family. In practice it has been our experience that the earlier communication approaches additional to speech are introduced, when they are indicated, the more readily they will be accepted and used realistically and appropriately. This applies particularly to the use of sophisticated technology involving, for example, eye gaze control. Clearly, the elements in decision-making with respect to the use of technology such as this include the availability of relevant resources, as well as the likelihood that the child with CP will become a reasonably independent and motivated adult with CP.

The other aspect of oromotor function that frequently requires consideration during adolescence is the safety and adequacy of chewing and swallowing, especially at a time in life when there is likely to be an adolescent growth spurt and associated increased nutritional and energy requirements. Not infrequently under these circumstances, weight gain tails off, something which can be seen both in adolescents who self-feed and in those who require to be fed. Moreover, if safe swallowing is somewhat precarious, there can be an increased risk of aspiration. In consequence, a minority of adolescents with CP require consideration of gastrostomy insertion for supplementary feeding at this time of their lives. The implications of this for long-term dependence are clear.

Research opportunities
From the scattering of evidence about transition to adulthood for young people with CP discussed in this chapter, it will be apparent that there is a yawning gap in our understanding of the issues. This opens up the possibility to chart new pathways in our understanding of the development of people with CP as they emerge from the childhood years and prepare for life as adults. Stewart (2009) and Sawyer and Macnee (2010) have presented ideas about how these issues might be approached.

We believe that there is a tremendous opportunity to apply modern thinking and conceptual frameworks to understand and support the transition of young people with neurodisabilities towards adulthood, and then to study whether and how these ideas 'work' when applied effectively. At the same time, we stress the importance of not simply conceiving of transitions as a specific phase of life that needs its own rules and procedures, but of seeing these processes as essential threads in the fabric of life.

We would hope that there would be discussions with families from the very early years of children's lives, in which long-term perspectives are identified and a path towards them is plotted. The impact of applying these concepts can, we believe, best be explored and validated with careful prospective longitudinal studies that explore whether ideas like those outlined in this chapter do in fact lead to more effective transitions and better adult outcomes. It is our hope that young clinicians and researchers will find these challenges stimulating and will seize the opportunities that cry out for attention.

References

Binks JA, Barden WS, Burke TA, Young NL (2007) What do we really know about the transition to adult-centered health care? A focus on cerebral palsy and spina bifida. *Arch Phys Med Rehabil* 88: 1064–73.

Dickinson HO, Parkinson KN, Ravens-Sieberer U et al. (2007) Self-reported quality of life of 8–12-year-old children with cerebral palsy: a cross-sectional European study. *Lancet* 369: 2171–8.

Hanna SE, Rosenbaum PL, Bartlett DJ et al. (2009) Stability and decline in gross motor function among children and youth with cerebral palsy aged 2 to 21 years. *Dev Med Child Neurol* 51: 295–302.

Law M, Baptiste S, Carswell A, McColl MA, Polagajko H, Pollock N (2005) *Canadian Occupational Performance Measure*, 4th edn. Ottawa, ON: CAOT Publications ACE.

Livingston MH, Stewart D, Rosenbaum PL, Russell DJ (2011) Exploring issues of participation among adolescents with cerebral palsy: what's important to them? *Phys Occup Ther Pediatr* 31: 275–87.

Nieuwenhuijsen C, Donkervoort M, Nieuwstraten W, Stam HJ, Roebroeck ME; Transition Research Group South West Netherlands (2009) Experienced problems of young adults with cerebral palsy: targets for rehabilitation care. *Arch Phys Med Rehabil* 90: 1891–7.

Roebroeck ME, Jahnsen R, Carona C, Kent RM, Chamberlain MA (2009) Adult outcomes and lifespan issues for people with childhood-onset physical disability. *Dev Med Child Neurol* 51: 670–8.

Rosenbaum P, Stewart D (2007) Perspectives on transitions: rethinking services for children and youth with developmental disabilities. *Arch Phys Med Rehabil* 88: 1080–2.

Sawyer SM, Macnee S (2010) Transition to adult health care for adolescents with spina bifida: research issues. *Dev Disabil Res Rev* 16: 60–5.

Stewart D (2009) Transition to adult services for young people with disabilities: current evidence to guide future research. *Dev Med Child Neurol* 51 (Suppl. 4): 169–73.

Stewart D, Law M, Rosenbaum PL, Willms D (2001) A qualitative study of the transition to adulthood for youth with physical disabilities. *Phys Occup Ther Pediatr* 21: 3–21.

Tieman B, Palisano RJ, Gracely EJ, Rosenbaum PL (2004) Gross motor capability and performance of mobility in children with cerebral palsy: a comparison across home, school, and outdoors/community settings. *Phys Ther* 84: 419–29.

Chapter 15

Adult functioning

Overview

As has been identified throughout this book, the idea of 'the adult with cerebral palsy (CP)' is still rather new, at least with respect to systematic studies of the lives and functioning of people in this population. It is sobering to realize that, based on epidemiological considerations, there should be approximately three times as many adults with CP as there are children and young people. This concluding chapter provides a summary of what is being discussed about four aspects of the lives of adults with CP. The themes include the health and social outcomes of adults with CP, some evidence of decline in function in the adult years and such information as is available on the quality of life of adults with CP. We also present what is known about life expectancy, recognizing that by its very nature such information is largely retrospective and hence potentially quite out of date.

At the end of the chapter we comment on the research challenges associated with obtaining accurate data on a population that has not been followed systematically. Finally, we identify a number of research opportunities that we hope will be taken up by colleagues across a range of fields and disciplines, so that the quantity and richness of what we know about adults with CP in the next decade and beyond will far outstrip the meagre number of currently available data.

Health and social outcomes in adult life

There is increasing interest in the 'outcomes' and well-being of adults with CP. Unfortunately, there remains a paucity of good information on the nature and quality of their lives, in part because CP has traditionally been considered a 'children's disorder', so there has been little systematic exploration of the lives of adults with CP. The knowledge that we do have is often biased by our awareness of the issues (almost always the difficulties) experienced by the relatively few adolescents and adults who may seek our advice. We almost certainly lack knowledge about the lives of people with CP who might be doing well but who, for a host of reasons, are outside our orbit.

Of course, the questions that parents ask about outcomes are often highly practical, yet may be posed with trepidation. These concern whether their child will be able to be mobile on their own, live independently, be 'productive', have a place in the community, marry and have a family. These are the same questions that most parents would want to know about their typically developing child's future, but in the case of children and young people with neurodisabilities, the questions are tinged with considerable anxiety. These concerns are fundamentally about 'outcomes' for which we have less information than we do about, for example, the impact of botulinum toxin on spastic muscles; however to parents and young people these bigger questions about the impact of the various outcomes on life may have far more importance.

Hitherto there have been no population studies that have provided an overall perspective on adults with CP, although a helpful summary of current knowledge and practice is provided by Haak et al. (2009). There are also a number of reviews and cross-sectional studies: those of Turk et al. (2001), Liptak and Accardo (2004) and Mesterman et al. (2010) provide data that are of interest. These are reviewed briefly here.

Liptak and Accardo (2004) noted that at the time of their paper, the employment rate for all adults with CP in the USA was 40%. They also made the point that in part this could be a reflection of there having been inadequate transition arrangements. Turk et al. (2001) found a very high rate of comorbid health factors in women with CP, making the point that these were present in spite of the fact that most if not all would have had extensive inputs in childhood. An implication of this report is that adults with CP receive different levels of health surveillance and care than are offered to children.

The study of Mesterman et al. (2010) examined the adult outcomes of an Israeli population who, as children, had been treated actively between 1975 and 2004. Of their respondents, 78% lived with their parents, 25% served in the army, 23% had a driver's licence and 23% worked in competitive employment. In this study, a large majority reported a high level of job satisfaction, although this was based on the relatively small proportion of people who actually had employment.

In addition, Wiegerink and her colleagues (2010) studied relationships and sexual activity in a Dutch population with CP. Among their findings was that levels of gross motor function were associated significantly with intercourse experience. Compared with an age-appropriate Dutch reference population, young adults with CP participated at a lower level in romantic relationships and sexual activities, but had equal sexual interest at the final assessment. They concluded that young ambulatory adults with CP had similar sexual interests and had increasing experiences with romantic relationships and sexual activities during the transition from late adolescence to young adulthood. However, in the age range 20–24 years, 41% of women (but only 19% of men) reported having a current romantic relationship.

There is a dearth of literature on the reproductive capacity of women with CP, but the clinical impression we gain is that childbearing is the exception rather than the rule. However, Winch et al. (1993) reviewed both the experiences of 22 women with CP who had been pregnant and the perinatal outcomes of their infants. It is relevant that 11 of the women were not reported to have any associated disabilities such as cognitive impairment or epilepsy and that none of the children appeared likely to have neurological disabilities.

It is important to report the caveat about these findings as noted by the authors themselves: 'The outcomes of this sample of mostly mildly to moderately affected women may not be representative of women with more severe CP. In addition, though our search was a systematic one, ascertainment bias may have affected the sample identified. There may have been incomplete coding of the diagnosis of CP by the staff who filled in the medical records. Mild cases of CP may have been either missed or not considered important by the clinicians. In the most severe cases, on the other hand, the diagnosis of CP may have been omitted from the coding, in favour of other diagnoses related to associated impairment (e.g. scoliosis or seizure disorder). We concentrated on tertiary obstetric services and it may be that more pregnant women with CP were cared for in community-level programs' (Winch et al. 1993, pp. 977–8). These interpretations of the data are consistent with the arguments about 'critical appraisal' made in Chapter 6 of this book.

It is also of interest that there are no reports detailing mental health disorders in adults with CP. Nevertheless, paediatric clinical experience, together with evidence of there being mental health vulnerability in populations with brain injury (Mortimer et al. 1985), makes it probable that, if sought, a whole range of mental health disorders would be recognized in adults with CP.

Decline in function
Cerebral palsy is an evolving disorder and its evolution continues into and throughout adult life. It is unsurprising, therefore, that some aspects of functioning decline with age and illness (as in people with ordinary functional capacity). This has been seen and reported particularly with respect to motor function.

Adults with CP are recognized as frequently developing musculoskeletal problems including fatigue, pain and a premature decline in mobility and function as they age. It also may well be that adults with CP are at risk of progressive impairments of other areas of function. It does however have to be emphasized that the available data are derived from limited samples that are not population based and are usually cross-sectional and potentially biased, as discussed above. It follows that caution is required before definitive generalizable conclusions can be drawn.

For some people with CP, decline in function begins in adolescence (Hanna et al. 2009). This is seen particularly in those who are more functionally affected and are at Gross Motor Function Classification System (GMFCS) levels III, IV and V. Cross-sectional studies, for example those of Murphy et al. (1995) and Bottos et al. (2001), have noted that significant percentages (up to 40%) of adults with CP who could walk in adolescence lost this ability over the course of the next two decades. It follows that a decline in motor function may frequently also affect those who are more motorically able earlier in their lives.

The causes of any decline require careful and individual assessment; they are likely to include increased body size following the adolescent growth spurt, decreased physical activity, osteoporosis, increased spasticity, hip and knee problems, pain and impaired balance. As is further detailed below, at least some of these challenges are probably 'secondary' disabilities that may to some extent be preventable and could benefit from appropriate anticipatory guidance and health-promoting interventions.

Decline in function may also be seen with respect to daily living activities. What limited evidence there is suggests that at an older age, functional deterioration with respect to these activities may occur. For example, Strauss et al. (2004) documented a loss of dressing skills in older people in California. There is also some anecdotal evidence that continence may deteriorate in some older people with CP (Middleton and O'Brien 2009).

The hypothetical possibility also exists that cognitive decline, dementia and significant mental health problems may be over-represented in older people with CP. This is based on the recognition that there may be a heightened risk of dementia in people with brain damage (Mortimer et al. 1985) and on the possibility of there being limited cognitive reserve in those with CP or other evidence of brain damage. However, there have been no population studies that support either of these propositions.

Quality of life issues

There are few quality of life (QoL) studies that use appropriate measures in adults with CP (see also Chapter 12). However, van der Slot and her colleagues (2010), in a study from the Netherlands on health-related QoL, concluded that a significant number of adults with bilateral spastic CP encountered difficulties in social participation and had a low perceived health-related QoL for physical functions. Higher general self-efficacy or a greater willingness to expend effort in achieving behaviour was related to better participation and a higher physical and mental health-related QoL. It is relevant that at least 60% of their sample had difficulties with mobility, recreation and housing and 44% had difficulty with personal care and employment. They perceived low health-related QoL for physical functions but not for cognitive functions.

Similarly, in a Norwegian study by Opheim et al. (2011), it was demonstrated that, in contrast to the general population, there was hardly any correlation between the number of pain sites and psychological health in adults with CP. The authors nevertheless made the point that improved pain management and evidence-based physiotherapy and rehabilitation programmes with a lifespan perspective should be recommended.

Although health-related QoL is adversely affected by factors such as immobility and pain, it is reasonable to hypothesize, based on studies of adolescents (Rosenbaum et al. 2007) and on the observations of Albrecht and Devlieger (1999), that other QoL factors in adults with CP will be largely independent of the degree of disability.

Life expectancy
As discussed below, it is now anticipated that the majority of people with CP will live through childhood and adolescence and well into adult life. A minority will, however, die in infancy and early childhood.

Against this background, life expectancy in CP is of interest for a number of reasons. These include the fact that, at the beginning of life, children who are known to have very severe brain abnormalities or a profound degree of brain damage are recognized as often having a very limited potential for survival. Children and their families affected in this way require appropriate counselling and inputs that recognize this reality, provide appropriate health and other counselling, and promote adaptation for the child and family as far as this is possible.

Clinical experience also suggests that, in general, those individuals who have the most severe disabilities but who nevertheless survive early infancy are likely to have overt constraints on their survival. There is, however, a world of difference between that general statement, which is based on epidemiological observations, and attempting to predict the probable survival time for any individual, even though this is a question that is often asked of treating paediatricians.

More generally, at a community level, planning for service provision for those with CP and other disabilities requires epidemiological information, including knowledge of probable life expectations. This applies not only to health services but also to social services and insurance providers.

It is against this background that we review here the current data on life expectation for people with CP.

The standard scientific definition of life expectancy is the average survival time of the members of a population. The life expectancy of a given individual is thus the average survival time of similar individuals in a large group of people who represent that individual's situation. It should therefore be clear that life expectancy does not predict the actual time that a specific individual will live, but provides an average value. In a specific situation that time could be much longer or shorter than an average life expectancy (Strauss et al. 2008).

There has been a continuing flow of publications on life expectation in CP. These include those of Blair et al. (2001), Hemming et al. (2006), Hutton and Pharoah (2002, 2006), Strauss et al. (2007) and Baird et al. (2011), as discussed below.

Strauss and his colleagues (2008) have recently brought relevant information on this subject up to date. Most of their data are derived from the population of disabled people who have received publicly funded services in California, USA. They have identified those within this population who have CP and, using a periodically updated client evaluation questionnaire, they have been able to identify their functional status with particular reference to mobility, hand function, methods of feeding, cognitive and linguistic functioning, and health status including epilepsy.

These authors have confirmed that in the long term for people with CP, the major quantifiable determinants of life expectation relate to their mobility and their nutritional and feeding status. It is unsurprising that, from the motor perspective, those who are immobile and unable to lift their heads in the prone position, and hence would be at GMFCS level V, have the shortest life expectations. This is especially the case for those who are also gastrostomy fed.

By contrast, adults with CP who can walk independently for at least 6m (i.e. those who would be at GMFCS levels I and II) have the longest predicted life expectations. This is illustrated in Table 15.1.

Some comments are required on the figures provided in this table. Firstly, the figures quoted refer to actual observed life expectations in California in 2008. These are empirical data based on a specific time period, place and service system. They do not refer to projected life expectations, which for uninjured individuals are currently some 10–12 years greater than the figures quoted. There is also likely to be a proportional increase in life expectancy for those with disabilities, which is supported by further work from Strauss and his colleagues (2007).

Secondly, it is of interest that neither Strauss et al. nor others have found that life expectancy correlates significantly with cognitive impairment unless this is of profound degree. In those situations it is likely that cognitive disabilities are confounded by other functional difficulties such as mobility and feeding restrictions, both of which, as indicated above, are known to have an independent relationship with survival.

Thirdly, the requirement of an individual to be tube fed (whether by gastrostomy or by an alternative route) must be considered as a marker both for overall severity of disability and of the individual's nutritional status. It is important to make clear, therefore, that it is not the need for tube feeding per se that shortens life expectancy. Indeed, it is likely that impaired nutritional status in a disabled child will correlate with an increased mortality risk and that satisfactory tube feeding will be associated with better nutrition, improved overall health and hence greater longevity.

Finally, it is relevant that even limited independent mobility, and the ability to sit unaided, confer a statistically increased life expectancy for people with CP.

Specific health factors cannot be examined in detail in epidemiological studies such as those of Strauss and his group, but they are nevertheless relevant. Indeed, the identified

Table 15.1
Mean life expectancy (additional years) by age and cohort. Published with permission from Strauss et al. (2008)

Sex/age (years)	Cannot lift head			Lifts head or chest			Rolls/sits, cannot walk			Walks unaided	General population
	TF	FBO	SF	TF	FBO	SF	TF	FBO	SF		
Female											
15	13	16	–	16	21	–	21	35	49	55	65.8
30	14	20	–	15	26	–	16	34	39	43	51.2
45	12	14	–	13	16	–	14	22	27	31	37.0
60	–	–	–	–	–	–	–	–	16	20	23.8
Male											
15	13	16	–	16	20	–	19	32	45	51	60.6
30	14	19	–	15	24	–	16	31	35	39	46.5
45	12	14	–	13	15	–	14	20	23	27	32.8
60	–	–	–	–	–	–	–	–	13	16	20.4

TF, tube fed; FBO, fed by others; SF, self-feeds.

causes of death in CP are most frequently chest and other infections. It follows that preventative measures to reduce the frequency and severity of these problems must have a prominence in overall management plans directed at preventing untimely death in people with CP.

Other health issues, such as nutritional status in people with CP and the optimal management of epilepsy, are also important. It has been shown that epilepsy acts as an independent, albeit minor, statistical constraint on life expectancy (Day et al. 2003), while so far as nutritional status is concerned, Brooks et al. (2011) have demonstrated, using the California database, that children at GMFCS levels III–V who are in the lowest 20% for weight have a statistically increased risk of early death.

Against this background, it is appropriate to speculate that the implementation and maintenance of multidisciplinary services for disabled children and their families, together with the provision of resourced care services, are relevant in providing not only optimal developmental inputs early in life but also preventative optimal health care. In this way such services may well contribute to the increase in life expectancy for disabled people.

It is important to remind readers once again that most of what we currently know about life expectancy, based on the best available evidence, is in some ways out of date and reflects the outcomes of processes and services offered many years ago. We believe that there is reason to be optimistic that appropriate prospective preventative programmes and services will alter and in fact improve the health and longevity of the current generation of children and young people with CP.

Perhaps the most important implication that can be derived from these figures is that in any population there will be more adults with CP than there are children with CP. For example, Hutton et al. (2006) have provided UK figures that indicate that the majority of children with three major disabilities survive into adult life; similarly, Strauss et al. (2007) state that 85% of severely disabled children live beyond the age of 14 years. In addition, Hemming et al. (2006) have reported that 85% of those who survive to the age of 20 years are still alive at 50.

We comment further on the significance of these prevalence figures below.

Intervention opportunities

For adults with CP who are mobile, maintaining their everyday mobility with support from informed carers, within the contexts of careful consideration of lifestyle changes and activity preferences, is the key element of any intervention programme. For some this entails a shift from self-reliance to increasing reliance on mobility aids and the assistance of others. These shifts may at times be based on personal choice. Whatever the case, the changes need to be made positively, with the emphasis being to identify whatever it is that offers the individual the best opportunities to take part in everyday life as independently as possible (O'Brien et al. 2009).

In addition, and because adults with CP tend to fatigue easily, periodic rests are advantageous. Other therapeutic approaches include effective weight management, and it is obvious that appropriate and effective pain management is of particular importance. It is also useful to make environmental adaptations, for example to a person's accommodation, when necessary.

Periodic use of the Functional Independence Measure (Balandin et al. 1997) may be helpful in assessing and planning for everyday activities in older people.

As well as these general measures, several specific therapeutic interventions can be helpful, many of which derive from paediatric practice. These include appropriately targeted physiotherapy and occupational therapy and low-impact physical exercise, for example swimming.

As with children, the use of baclofen and botulinum toxin injections can be helpful when spasticity is causing pain and limitation of movement in adults with CP. The use of intrathecal baclofen is recognized as being helpful in carefully selected individuals (Krach 2009), and there is suggestive evidence that its use may improve life expectancy (Krach et al. 2010).

For more severely affected non-ambulatory individuals – for example those with persisting pain, difficulty in maintaining satisfactory supported seating or difficulties with perineal access – orthopaedic surgical procedures such as excision, relocation or replacement of hip joints may be indicated and useful. In the ambulatory patient, caution is required with respect to offering orthopaedic surgery as it is recognized that many adults do not rehabilitate as well or as quickly as children do. Because of this reality, orthopaedic interventions are usually limited to dealing with degenerative joint disease with joint replacement if possible and relatively minor interventions that will not require a prolonged period of non-weight-bearing post-operatively.

A further specific area that frequently requires attention is continence management, especially when continence control deteriorates. Here the key to management is to identify, wherever possible, the cause of loss of continence, for example constipation or a urinary tract infection, and of course to institute appropriate management. As always, preventative interventions are the preferred approach to management.

Other health interventions that are relevant and can maintain or promote continuing independence include the recognition and treatment of chest and other infections, maintenance of dental hygiene and scrupulous skin care.

Conclusions
The appropriate conclusions to be drawn are that in the large population of adults with CP, those who are likely to be most independent will generally have good health, preserved cognition and few mobility limitations. By contrast, poor health, cognitive impairment and relative immobility are factors that are likely to correlate with

long-term dependence. It follows that in childhood and during transition to adult life, realistic long-term planning and provision are not only required but should also be, at least potentially, achievable.

References

Albrecht GL, Devlieger PJ (1999) The disability paradox: high quality of life against all odds. *Soc Sci Med* 48: 977–88.

Baird G, Allen E, Srutton D et al. (2011) Mortality from 1 – 16–18 in bilateral cerebral palsy. *Arch Dis Child* 96: 1077–81.

Balandin S, Alexander B, Hoffman D (1997) Use of the Functional Independence Measure to assess adults with cerebral palsy: an exploratory report. *J Appl Res Intellect Disabil* 10: 323–32.

Blair E, Watson L, Badawi N, Stanley FJ (2001) Life expectancy among people with cerebral palsy in Western Australia. *Dev Med Child Neurol* 43: 508–15.

Bottos M, Feliciangeli A, Sciuto L, Gericke C, Vianello A (2001) Functional status of adults with cerebral palsy and implications for treatment of children. *Dev Med Child Neurol* 43: 516–28.

Brooks J, Day S, Shavelle R, Strauss D (2011) Low weight, morbidity, and mortality in children with cerebral palsy: new clinical growth charts. *Pediatrics* 129: e299–e307.

Day S, Strauss D, Shavelle R, Wu YW (2003) Excess mortality in remote symptomatic epilepsy. *J Ins Med* 35: 15–20.

Haak P, Lenski M, Hidecker MJ, Li M, Paneth N (2009) Cerebral palsy and aging. *Dev Med Child Neurol* 51 (Suppl. 4): 16–23.

Hanna SE, Rosenbaum PL, Bartlett DJ et al. (2009) Stability and decline in gross motor function among children and youth with cerebral palsy aged 2 to 21 years. *Dev Med Child Neurol* 51: 295–302.

Hemming K, Hutton JL, Pharoah PO (2006) Long-term survival for a cohort of adults with cerebral palsy. *Dev Med Child Neurol* 48: 90–5.

Hutton JL, Pharoah POD (2002) Effects of cognitive, motor, and sensory disabilities on survival in cerebral palsy. *Arch Dis Child* 86: 84–9.

Hutton JL, Pharoah POD (2006) Life expectancy in severe cerebral palsy. *Arch Dis Child*, 91:254–8.

Krach LE (2009) Intrathecal baclofen use in adults with cerebral palsy. *Dev Med Child Neurol* 51 (Suppl. 4): 106–12.

Krach LE, Kriel RL, Day SM, Strauss DJ (2010) Survival of individuals with cerebral palsy receiving continuous intrathecal baclofen treatment: a matched-cohort study. *Dev Med Child Neurol* 52: 672–6.

Liptak GS, Accardo PJ (2004) Health and social outcomes of children with cerebral palsy. *Paediatrics* 52: S36–41.

Mesterman R, Leitner Y, Yifat R et al. (2010) Cerebral palsy – long-term medical, functional, educational, and psychosocial outcomes. *J Child Neurol* 25: 36–42.

Middleton C, O'Brien G (2009) Living with ageing in developmental disability. In: O'Brien G, Rosenbloom L, editors. *Developmental Disability and Aging*. London: Mac Keith Press.

Mortimer JA, French LR, Hutton JT, Schuman LM (1985) Head injury as a risk factor for Alzheimer's disease. *Neurology* 35: 264–7.

Murphy KP, Molnar GE, Lankasky K (1995) Medical and functional status of adults with cerebral palsy. *Dev Med Child Neurol* 37: 1075–84.

O'Brien G, Bass A, Rosenbloom L (2009) Cerebral palsy and aging. In: O'Brien G, Rosenbloom L, editors. *Developmental Disability and Aging*. London: Mac Keith Press.

Opheim A, Jahnsen R, Olsson E, Stanghelle JK (2011) Physical and mental components of health-related quality of life and musculoskeletal pain sites over seven years in adults with spastic cerebral palsy. *J Rehabil Med* 43: 382–7.

Rosenbaum PL, Livingston MH, Palisano RJ, Galuppi BE, Russell DJ (2007) Quality of life and health-related quality of life of adolescents with cerebral palsy. *Dev Med Child Neurol* 49: 516–21.

van der Slot WMA, Nieuwenhuijsen C, van den Berg-Emons RJG, Wensink-Boonstra AE, Stam HJ, Roebroeck ME (2010) Participation and health-related quality of life in adults with spastic bilateral cerebral palsy and the role of self-efficacy. *Rehabil Med* 42: 528–35.

Strauss DJ, Ojdana KA, Shavelle RM, Rosenbloom L (2004) Decline in function and life expectancy of older persons with cerebral palsy. *NeuroRehabilitation* 19: 69–78.

Strauss DJ, Shavelle RM, Reynolds RJ, Rosenbloom L, Day SM (2007) Survival in cerebral palsy in the last 20 years: Signs of improvement? *Dev Med Child Neurol* 49: 86–92.

Strauss DJ, Shavelle RM, Rosenbloom L, Brooks JC (2008) Life expectancy in cerebral palsy: An update. *Dev Med Child Neurol* 50: 487–93.

Turk MA, Scandale J, Rosenbaum PF, Weber RJ (2001) The health of women with cerebral palsy. *Phys Med Rehabil Clin N Am* 12: 153–68.

Wiegerink DJ, Stam HJ, Gorter JW, Cohen-Kettenis PT, Roebroeck ME, Transition Research Group Southwest Netherlands (2010) Development of romantic relationships and sexual activity in young adults with cerebral palsy: a longitudinal study. *Arch Phys Med Rehabil* 91: 1423–8.

Winch R, Bengston L, McLaughlin J, Fitzsimmons J, Budden S (1993) Women with cerebral palsy: obstetric experience and neonatal outcome. *Dev Med Child Neurol* 35: 974–82.

Glossary

Acidosis An increase in the level of acidity in the blood or other body tissues. In the case of the newborn infant, this can arise when there are limitations in oxygen supply.

Adjunctive In the context of medial treatments, adjunctive interventions are those that are added to the standard approaches.

Aetiological Causal.

Anencephaly Absence of a large part of the brain, a condition that develops early in fetal life and is not compatible with long-term survival after birth.

Antiphospholipid syndrome A condition of increased coagulability of the blood that is associated with pregnancy-related complications such as miscarriages and preterm delivery.

Apgar score A clinical assessment of a newborn infant's adjustment to being out of the womb, usually assessed at 1 and 5 minutes after delivery.

Ataxia Impaired coordination of movement and motor control in the absence of muscle weakness. Ataxia normally implies impairment of function of the cerebellum (see below).

Ataxia–telangiectasia A rare inherited neurodegenerative condition that affects the body's coordination of motor function and its immune system.

Athetosis Involuntary, writhing movements of the fingers, arms, legs and neck. Usually seen in extrapyramidal motor disorders (see below).

Babinski response   Abnormal extensor (upwards) reflex movements of the big toes when the outer borders of the feet are stroked.

Baclofen   A drug used to treat spasticity; it can be administered by mouth or delivered directly into the space around the spinal cord (at much lower doses than are needed when the drug is used orally). This is termed intrathecal administration.

Basal ganglia   Groups of nerve cells in the brain that function, among other things, to influence voluntary motor control and can be damaged by a variety of problems in the newborn period, including severe oxygen restriction to the brain. They are a component of the extrapyramidal motor system.

Benzodiazepines   A group of drugs that affect the chemical activity of a specific neurotransmitter in the brain and have, among their many effects, muscle-relaxing action.

Biphosphonates   A group of drugs that prevent the loss of bone mass and are used to treat osteoporosis and other conditions of bone chemistry.

Botulinum toxin   A protein produced by a bacterium that, in sufficient concentrations, causes 'botulism', a serious and often fatal poisoning; used in small doses by injection to produce a temporary (3–6mo) weakening of spastic muscles.

Cardiotocography   A technical means of recording (*graphy*) the fetal heartbeat (*cardio*) and uterine contractions (*toco*) during pregnancy and labour.

Cerebellum   A region of the hindbrain that is concerned primarily with balance and coordination functions.

Cerebral perfusion   The flow of blood through the vessels of the brain to supply fresh oxygenated blood from the heart (through the arteries) and remove unoxygenated blood back to the heart (through the veins).

Choreoathetosis   See athetosis.

Chorioamnionitis   An inflammation of the membranes (chorion and amnion) that surround the fetus while in the womb, usually caused by bacteria and potentially leading to serious health risks to both the infant and the mother.

Cognitive impairment   Used synonymously for mental retardation.

Comorbid   Refers to the presence of one or more disorders (or diseases) in addition to a primary disease or disorder, or the effect of such additional disorders or diseases.

Corticobulbar tract   Carries information from the cerebral cortex to the brainstem.

Corticospinal tract A collection of motor fibres that conduct impulses from the motor cortex in the cerebral hemispheres to the spinal cord.

Cytomegalovirus (also called CMV) One of a group of viruses that can infect a fetus in utero and, depending on the timing of the infection in pregnancy, cause permanent damage to the brain with associated neurodevelopmental disabilities.

Developmental retardation Indicates developmental delay, which may be permanent, affecting some or all parameters of development. Tends to be used in young children.

Diplegia In cerebral palsy, this term is used to refer to functional impairment of the legs that is more severe than functional impairment of the upper extremities.

Dyskinetic Abnormal patterns of posture and/or movement, associated with involuntary, uncontrolled, recurring, occasionally stereotyped movement patterns. Includes athetoid and choreoathetoid involuntary movements.

Dysmorphic A medical term referring to a difference of body structure that may be suggestive of a congenital disorder, genetic syndrome or birth defect.

Dysphagia Difficulty in swallowing.

Dysphasia Partial or complete impairment of the ability to communicate resulting from brain injury.

Dystocia An abnormal labour or difficult childbirth arising from poorly coordinated uterine activity, an abnormal position of the infant as it is emerging from the birth canal, structural differences in the infant (such as an enlarged head) or problems in the structure of the birth canal.

Dystonia Involuntary fluctuations of muscle tone due to extrapyramidal motor dysfunction. Often associated with involuntary athetoid movements.

Encephalopathy A general terms that refers to disorder or disease of the central nervous system.

Epidemiology The study of health events, health characteristics or health-determinant patterns in a population.

Eponym The name of a person or thing, whether real or fictitious, after which a particular place, tribe, era, discovery or other item is named or thought to be named. In medicine this refers to diseases or conditions.

Excitotoxicity A pathological process in which nerve cells are damaged or killed by excess stimulation by chemicals (neurotransmitters).

Extrapyramidal system   A neural network that is part of the motor system that causes involuntary reflexes and movement and modulation of movement (i.e. coordination). The system is called 'extrapyramidal' to distinguish it from the tracts of the motor cortex that reach their targets by travelling through the 'pyramids' of the medulla.

Focal infarction   Refers to localized tissue death (necrosis) caused by a local lack of oxygen owing to obstruction of the tissue's blood supply; the resulting lesion is referred to as an infarct.

Germinal matrix   A highly cellular and highly vascularized region in the brain from which cells migrate out during brain development; the source of both neurones and glial cells; most active between 8 and 28 weeks' gestation. It is a fragile portion of the brain that may be damaged, leading to an intracranial haemorrhage known as a germinal matrix haemorrhage.

Globus pallidus   A part of the basal ganglia (see above).

Glutamate   A chemical neurotransmitter that is both an essential brain chemical and one that, in excess amounts, can be toxic to the brain.

Glutaric aciduria   An inherited disorder in which the body is unable to metabolize certain amino acids, leading to processes that cause damage to the brain, in particular to the basal ganglia (see above).

Goniometer   A hand-held device to measure joint angles.

Gyrus/gyri   A ridge(s) on the surface of the brain.

Habilitative   As used in this book, the term refers to 'development' – the promotion of functional status in any aspects of a child's life (in distinction to 'rehabilitative' efforts, which imply a return to a former state of function).

Hemiplegia   A term used to describe functional motor impairment on one side of the body (as may be seen in an adult after a stroke or in a child after impairment of the brain on the side of the body opposite to the functional limitation).

Hemimegalencephaly   A rare abnormality in the development of the brain whereby half of the brain is abnormally enlarged, usually leading to seizures and impaired development.

Hemiparesis   See hemiplegia above.

Hemispherectomy   Surgical removal of half (*hemi*) of the brain.

Heterodox   Not in accordance with established or accepted approaches (opposite of 'orthodox').

Heterotopias   The formation and presence of tissue in a part of the body where its presence is abnormal.

Hippocampal   Referring to the 'hippocampus', an important part of the 'limbic' system of the brain involved in memory.

Hippotherapy   A form of developmental therapy in which a therapist uses the characteristic movements of a horse to provide motor and sensory input for the rider.

Hydrocephalus   A build-up of fluid inside the skull, due to a problem with the flow of the fluid within and surrounding the brain, that leads to brain swelling.

Hyperbilirubinaemia   A condition in which there is an excess of bilirubin, produced when red blood cells (and haemoglobin) are broken down chemically. Excess bilirubin causes jaundice and in the susceptible newborn infant can lead to brain damage.

Hypertonus/hypertonic   A state of excess tone in muscles, referring to the amount of contraction that remains in a muscle when it is not actively working.

Hypocarbia   The condition of having an abnormally low level of carbon dioxide in the circulating blood.

Hypothyroidism   A condition in which the thyroid gland in the neck does not make enough thyroid hormone. Infants born to hypothyroid mothers, or with an inadequate capacity to make thyroid hormone, may develop cognitive impairment, cerebral palsy and deafness.

Intrapartum   During (*intra*) the process of delivery (*parturition*).

Ischaemia   A restriction in blood supply to tissues, causing a shortage of oxygen and glucose needed for cellular metabolism (to keep tissue alive).

Kernicterus   Damage to centres of the infant brain caused by excess levels of bilirubin for any of a number of reasons (see also hyperbilirubinaemia).

Ketogenic diet   A special diet used to treat some cases of refractory epilepsy (see below); the diet is very rich in fatty foods, causing the body to make high levels of ketones that often reduce the frequency of seizures.

Learning difficulties/impairment   Used synonymously for mental retardation.

Lentiform nuclei   Part of the basal ganglia of the brain (see basal ganglia).

Lesch–Nyhan syndrome   An inborn error of body chemistry due to an enzyme defect. A cause of brain damage.

Lissencephaly   Literally *smooth brain*, a rare disorder of brain formation caused by defective neuronal migration during the twelfth to twenty-fourth week of gestation, resulting in a lack of development of brain folds (gyri) and grooves.

Maternal rhesus iso-immunization   Incompatibility between blood groups of mother and fetus, as a result of which the mother's immune system creates antibodies to the fetus's blood and causes the blood to break down, leading to hyperbilirubinaemia (see above) and possibly to kernicterus (see above).

Mental retardation   This term is used in DSM IV classification system to describe significant cognitive impairment.

Microcephaly   Abnormally small head growth, usually associated with (caused by) poor brain development.

Myelopathy   Any pathology of the spinal cord, whether caused by inflammation, infection, trauma or poor blood supply.

Neuropathology   The study of disease of nervous system tissue.

NICU   Neonatal intensive care unit (in some countries these are called special care baby units), in which very sick and preterm infants are cared for after delivery.

Nystagmus   A condition of involuntary (jiggly) eye movement, acquired in infancy or later in life, that may result in reduced or limited vision.

Oromotor   Refers to the muscular control and coordination of the muscles of the face, lips and tongue needed for eating and speaking.

Parenchyma   The functional parts of an organ of the body (in contrast to the stroma, which refers to the connective tissues [structure] of the organ).

Perfusion failure   A problem with the adequate delivery of blood (containing oxygen and nutrients) to body tissues.

Periventricular   Around (*peri*) the ventricular fluid spaces in the brain.

Periventricular leukomalacia   A form of white-matter ('leuko') brain injury, characterized by damage to the brain's white matter near the lateral ventricles.

Phenomenological   As used in this book, this concept refers to the idea that many neurodevelopmental conditions (such as cerebral palsy) are conceptually linked by a set of defined characteristics rather than being specific and discrete diseases or disorders.

PKU (phenylketonuria)   A recessively inherited genetic condition in which the absence of a specific chemical factor (an enzyme) causes the body to build up high concentrations of 'phenylketones' that are damaging to brain tissue.

Placental abruption   A complication of pregnancy in which the placenta separates prematurely from the wall of the uterus, leading to deprivation of fetal oxygen supply and putting the unborn infant at risk of brain damage.

Plasticity   How entire brain structures, and the brain itself, can change based on new experience.

Polymicrogyria   A developmental malformation of the human brain characterized by an excessive number of small convolutions (gyri) on the surface of the brain; the whole surface (generalized) or parts of the surface (focal) can be affected.

Premorbid   Occurring or existing before the occurrence of physical disease or emotional illness.

Protean   Extremely variable.

Pyramidal tracts   Both the *corticospinal* and *corticobulbar tracts*.

Quadriplegia (Latin)/tetraplegia (Greek)   Partial or total loss of use of all limbs and torso.

Refractory epilepsy/seizures   Epilepsy that is very hard to control and is poorly responsive ('refractory') to the usual treatment approaches.

Rett syndrome   A genetic disorder, usually only affecting females, that is a cause of brain damage and malfunction.

Schizencephaly   A form of brain maldevelopment in which there is a cleft in the brain tissue associated with varying degrees of brain damage and malfunction.

Scoliosis   Abnormal curvature of the spine; may be progressive.

Sequelae   Pathological conditions that result from a disease or injury.

Severe learning difficulties/impairment   Used synonymously for mental retardation.

Spasticity   Increased muscle tone producing apperception of stiffness. Technically spastic muscles have a velocity-dependent resistance to stretch.

Thalamus/thalamic   Structures within the human brain situated between the cerebral hemispheres and midbrain; function includes relaying sensory and motor signals to the cerebral cortex, along with the regulation of consciousness, sleep and alertness.

Thrombophilic   An abnormal tendency for the blood to clot, increasing the risk of blood clots in the vessels.

Topographic   Referring to the distribution of cerebral palsy in the body (one side, hemiplegia; predominant leg involvement, diplegia; whole body involvement, quadriplegia/tetraplegia).

Trisomy 21   Down syndrome.

Videofluoroscopy   Radiological investigation of swallowing capacity.

Appendices

CanChild Centre for Childhood Disability Research
Institute for Applied Health Sciences, McMaster University,
1400 Main Street West, Room 408, Hamilton, ON, Canada L8S 1C7
Tel: 905-525-9140 ext. 27850 Fax: 905-522-6095
E-mail: canchild@mcmaster.ca Website: www.canchild.ca

GMFCS – E & R
Gross Motor Function Classification System
Expanded and Revised

GMFCS - E & R © Robert Palisano, Peter Rosenbaum, Doreen Bartlett, Michael Livingston, 2007
CanChild Centre for Childhood Disability Research, McMaster University

GMFCS © Robert Palisano, Peter Rosenbaum, Stephen Walter, Dianne Russell, Ellen Wood, Barbara Galuppi, 1997
CanChild Centre for Childhood Disability Research, McMaster University
(Reference: Dev Med Child Neurol 1997;39:214-223)

INTRODUCTION & USER INSTRUCTIONS

The Gross Motor Function Classification System (GMFCS) for cerebral palsy is based on self-initiated movement, with emphasis on sitting, transfers, and mobility. When defining a five-level classification system, our primary criterion has been that the distinctions between levels must be meaningful in daily life. Distinctions are based on functional limitations, the need for hand-held mobility devices (such as walkers, crutches, or canes) or wheeled mobility, and to a much lesser extent, quality of movement. The distinctions between Levels I and II are not as pronounced as the distinctions between the other levels, particularly for infants less than 2 years of age.

The expanded GMFCS (2007) includes an age band for youth 12 to 18 years of age and emphasizes the concepts inherent in the World Health Organization's International Classification of Functioning, Disability and Health (ICF). We encourage users to be aware of the impact that **environmental** and **personal** factors may have on what children and youth are observed or reported to do. The focus of the GMFCS is on determining which level best represents the **child's or youth's present abilities and limitations in gross motor function**. Emphasis is on usual **performance** in home, school, and community settings (i.e., what they do), rather than what they are known to be able to do at their best (capability). It is therefore important to classify current performance in gross motor function and not to include judgments about the quality of movement or prognosis for improvement.

The title for each level is the method of mobility that is most characteristic of performance after 6 years of age. The descriptions of functional abilities and limitations for each age band are broad and are not intended to describe all aspects of the function of individual children/youth. For example, an infant with hemiplegia who is unable to crawl on his or her hands and knees, but otherwise fits the description of Level I (i.e., can pull to stand and walk), would be classified in Level I. The scale is ordinal, with no intent that the distances between levels be considered equal or that children and youth with cerebral palsy are equally distributed across the five levels. A summary of the distinctions between each pair of levels is provided to assist in determining the level that most closely resembles a child's/youth's current gross motor function.

We recognize that the manifestations of gross motor function are dependent on age, especially during infancy and early childhood. For each level, separate descriptions are provided in several age bands. Children below age 2 should be considered at their corrected age if they were premature. The descriptions for the 6 to 12 year and 12 to18 year age bands reflect the potential impact of environment factors (e.g., distances in school and community) and personal factors (e.g., energy demands and social preferences) on methods of mobility.

An effort has been made to emphasize abilities rather than limitations. Thus, as a general principle, the gross motor function of children and youth who are able to perform the functions described in any particular level will probably be classified at or above that level of function; in contrast, the gross motor function of children and youth who cannot perform the functions of a particular level should be classified below that level of function.

Available at http://motorgrowth.canchild.ca/en/GMFCS/resources/GMFCS-ER.pdf.

OPERATIONAL DEFINITIONS

Body support walker – A mobility device that supports the pelvis and trunk. The child/youth is physically positioned in the walker by another person.

Hand-held mobility device – Canes, crutches, and anterior and posterior walkers that do not support the trunk during walking.

Physical assistance – Another person manually assists the child/youth to move.

Powered mobility – The child/youth actively controls the joystick or electrical switch that enables independent mobility. The mobility base may be a wheelchair, scooter or other type of powered mobility device.

Self-propels manual wheelchair – The child/youth actively uses arms and hands or feet to propel the wheels and move.

Transported – A person manually pushes a mobility device (e.g., wheelchair, stroller, or pram) to move the child/youth from one place to another.

Walks – Unless otherwise specified indicates no physical assistance from another person or any use of a hand-held mobility device. An orthosis (i.e., brace or splint) may be worn.

Wheeled mobility – Refers to any type of device with wheels that enables movement (e.g., stroller, manual wheelchair, or powered wheelchair).

GENERAL HEADINGS FOR EACH LEVEL

LEVEL I	-	Walks without Limitations
LEVEL II	-	Walks with Limitations
LEVEL III	-	Walks Using a Hand-Held Mobility Device
LEVEL IV	-	Self-Mobility with Limitations; May Use Powered Mobility
LEVEL V	-	Transported in a Manual Wheelchair

DISTINCTIONS BETWEEN LEVELS

Distinctions Between Levels I and II - Compared with children and youth in Level I, children and youth in Level II have limitations walking long distances and balancing; may need a hand-held mobility device when first learning to walk; may use wheeled mobility when traveling long distances outdoors and in the community; require the use of a railing to walk up and down stairs; and are not as capable of running and jumping.

Distinctions Between Levels II and III - Children and youth in Level II are capable of walking without a hand-held mobility device after age 4 (although they may choose to use one at times). Children and youth in Level III need a hand-held mobility device to walk indoors and use wheeled mobility outdoors and in the community.

Distinctions Between Levels III and IV - Children and youth in Level III sit on their own or require at most limited external support to sit, are more independent in standing transfers, and walk with a hand-held mobility device. Children and youth in Level IV function in sitting (usually supported) but self-mobility is limited. Children and youth in Level IV are more likely to be transported in a manual wheelchair or use powered mobility.

Distinctions Between Levels IV and V - Children and youth in Level V have severe limitations in head and trunk control and require extensive assisted technology and physical assistance. Self-mobility is achieved only if the child/youth can learn how to operate a powered wheelchair.

Gross Motor Function Classification System – Expanded and Revised (GMFCS – E & R)

BEFORE 2ND BIRTHDAY

LEVEL I: Infants move in and out of sitting and floor sit with both hands free to manipulate objects. Infants crawl on hands and knees, pull to stand and take steps holding on to furniture. Infants walk between 18 months and 2 years of age without the need for any assistive mobility device.

LEVEL II: Infants maintain floor sitting but may need to use their hands for support to maintain balance. Infants creep on their stomach or crawl on hands and knees. Infants may pull to stand and take steps holding on to furniture.

LEVEL III: Infants maintain floor sitting when the low back is supported. Infants roll and creep forward on their stomachs.

LEVEL IV: Infants have head control but trunk support is required for floor sitting. Infants can roll to supine and may roll to prone.

LEVEL V: Physical impairments limit voluntary control of movement. Infants are unable to maintain antigravity head and trunk postures in prone and sitting. Infants require adult assistance to roll.

BETWEEN 2ND AND 4TH BIRTHDAY

LEVEL I: Children floor sit with both hands free to manipulate objects. Movements in and out of floor sitting and standing are performed without adult assistance. Children walk as the preferred method of mobility without the need for any assistive mobility device.

LEVEL II: Children floor sit but may have difficulty with balance when both hands are free to manipulate objects. Movements in and out of sitting are performed without adult assistance. Children pull to stand on a stable surface. Children crawl on hands and knees with a reciprocal pattern, cruise holding onto furniture and walk using an assistive mobility device as preferred methods of mobility.

LEVEL III: Children maintain floor sitting often by "W-sitting" (sitting between flexed and internally rotated hips and knees) and may require adult assistance to assume sitting. Children creep on their stomach or crawl on hands and knees (often without reciprocal leg movements) as their primary methods of self-mobility. Children may pull to stand on a stable surface and cruise short distances. Children may walk short distances indoors using a hand-held mobility device (walker) and adult assistance for steering and turning.

LEVEL IV: Children floor sit when placed, but are unable to maintain alignment and balance without use of their hands for support. Children frequently require adaptive equipment for sitting and standing. Self-mobility for short distances (within a room) is achieved through rolling, creeping on stomach, or crawling on hands and knees without reciprocal leg movement.

LEVEL V: Physical impairments restrict voluntary control of movement and the ability to maintain antigravity head and trunk postures. All areas of motor function are limited. Functional limitations in sitting and standing are not fully compensated for through the use of adaptive equipment and assistive technology. At Level V, children have no means of independent movement and are transported. Some children achieve self-mobility using a powered wheelchair with extensive adaptations.

BETWEEN 4TH AND 6TH BIRTHDAY

LEVEL I: Children get into and out of, and sit in, a chair without the need for hand support. Children move from the floor and from chair sitting to standing without the need for objects for support. Children walk indoors and outdoors, and climb stairs. Emerging ability to run and jump.

LEVEL II: Children sit in a chair with both hands free to manipulate objects. Children move from the floor to standing and from chair sitting to standing but often require a stable surface to push or pull up on with their arms. Children walk without the need for a hand-held mobility device indoors and for short distances on level surfaces outdoors. Children climb stairs holding onto a railing but are unable to run or jump.

LEVEL III: Children sit on a regular chair but may require pelvic or trunk support to maximize hand function. Children move in and out of chair sitting using a stable surface to push on or pull up with their arms. Children walk with a hand-held mobility device on level surfaces and climb stairs with assistance from an adult. Children frequently are transported when traveling for long distances or outdoors on uneven terrain.

LEVEL IV: Children sit on a chair but need adaptive seating for trunk control and to maximize hand function. Children move in and out of chair sitting with assistance from an adult or a stable surface to push or pull up on with their arms. Children may at best walk short distances with a walker and adult supervision but have difficulty turning and maintaining balance on uneven surfaces. Children are transported in the community. Children may achieve self-mobility using a powered wheelchair.

LEVEL V: Physical impairments restrict voluntary control of movement and the ability to maintain antigravity head and trunk postures. All areas of motor function are limited. Functional limitations in sitting and standing are not fully compensated for through the use of adaptive equipment and assistive technology. At Level V, children have no means of independent movement and are transported. Some children achieve self-mobility using a powered wheelchair with extensive adaptations.

BETWEEN 6TH AND 12TH BIRTHDAY

Level I: Children walk at home, school, outdoors, and in the community. Children are able to walk up and down curbs without physical assistance and stairs without the use of a railing. Children perform gross motor skills such as running and jumping but speed, balance, and coordination are limited. Children may participate in physical activities and sports depending on personal choices and environmental factors.

Level II: Children walk in most settings. Children may experience difficulty walking long distances and balancing on uneven terrain, inclines, in crowded areas, confined spaces or when carrying objects. Children walk up and down stairs holding onto a railing or with physical assistance if there is no railing. Outdoors and in the community, children may walk with physical assistance, a hand-held mobility device, or use wheeled mobility when traveling long distances. Children have at best only minimal ability to perform gross motor skills such as running and jumping. Limitations in performance of gross motor skills may necessitate adaptations to enable participation in physical activities and sports.

Level III: Children walk using a hand-held mobility device in most indoor settings. When seated, children may require a seat belt for pelvic alignment and balance. Sit-to-stand and floor-to-stand transfers require physical assistance of a person or support surface. When traveling long distances, children use some form of wheeled mobility. Children may walk up and down stairs holding onto a railing with supervision or physical assistance. Limitations in walking may necessitate adaptations to enable participation in physical activities and sports including self-propelling a manual wheelchair or powered mobility.

Level IV: Children use methods of mobility that require physical assistance or powered mobility in most settings. Children require adaptive seating for trunk and pelvic control and physical assistance for most transfers. At home, children use floor mobility (roll, creep, or crawl), walk short distances with physical assistance, or use powered mobility. When positioned, children may use a body support walker at home or school. At school, outdoors, and in the community, children are transported in a manual wheelchair or use powered mobility. Limitations in mobility necessitate adaptations to enable participation in physical activities and sports, including physical assistance and/or powered mobility.

Level V: Children are transported in a manual wheelchair in all settings. Children are limited in their ability to maintain antigravity head and trunk postures and control arm and leg movements. Assistive technology is used to improve head alignment, seating, standing, and and/or mobility but limitations are not fully compensated by equipment. Transfers require complete physical assistance of an adult. At home, children may move short distances on the floor or may be carried by an adult. Children may achieve self-mobility using powered mobility with extensive adaptations for seating and control access. Limitations in mobility necessitate adaptations to enable participation in physical activities and sports including physical assistance and using powered mobility.

BETWEEN 12TH AND 18TH BIRTHDAY

Level I: Youth walk at home, school, outdoors, and in the community. Youth are able to walk up and down curbs without physical assistance and stairs without the use of a railing. Youth perform gross motor skills such as running and jumping but speed, balance, and coordination are limited. Youth may participate in physical activities and sports depending on personal choices and environmental factors.

Level II: Youth walk in most settings. Environmental factors (such as uneven terrain, inclines, long distances, time demands, weather, and peer acceptability) and personal preference influence mobility choices. At school or work, youth may walk using a hand-held mobility device for safety. Outdoors and in the community, youth may use wheeled mobility when traveling long distances. Youth walk up and down stairs holding a railing or with physical assistance if there is no railing. Limitations in performance of gross motor skills may necessitate adaptations to enable participation in physical activities and sports.

Level III: Youth are capable of walking using a hand-held mobility device. Compared to individuals in other levels, youth in Level III demonstrate more variability in methods of mobility depending on physical ability and environmental and personal factors. When seated, youth may require a seat belt for pelvic alignment and balance. Sit-to-stand and floor-to-stand transfers require physical assistance from a person or support surface. At school, youth may self-propel a manual wheelchair or use powered mobility. Outdoors and in the community, youth are transported in a wheelchair or use powered mobility. Youth may walk up and down stairs holding onto a railing with supervision or physical assistance. Limitations in walking may necessitate adaptations to enable participation in physical activities and sports including self-propelling a manual wheelchair or powered mobility.

Level IV: Youth use wheeled mobility in most settings. Youth require adaptive seating for pelvic and trunk control. Physical assistance from 1 or 2 persons is required for transfers. Youth may support weight with their legs to assist with standing transfers. Indoors, youth may walk short distances with physical assistance, use wheeled mobility, or, when positioned, use a body support walker. Youth are physically capable of operating a powered wheelchair. When a powered wheelchair is not feasible or available, youth are transported in a manual wheelchair. Limitations in mobility necessitate adaptations to enable participation in physical activities and sports, including physical assistance and/or powered mobility.

Level V: Youth are transported in a manual wheelchair in all settings. Youth are limited in their ability to maintain antigravity head and trunk postures and control arm and leg movements. Assistive technology is used to improve head alignment, seating, standing, and mobility but limitations are not fully compensated by equipment. Physical assistance from 1 or 2 persons or a mechanical lift is required for transfers. Youth may achieve self-mobility using powered mobility with extensive adaptations for seating and control access. Limitations in mobility necessitate adaptations to enable participation in physical activities and sports including physical assistance and using powered mobility.

Appendix II

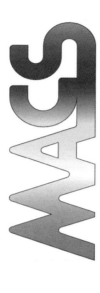

Manual Ability Classification System for Children with Cerebral Palsy
4-18 years

2005, updated 2010

MACS classifies how children with cerebral palsy use their hands to handle objects in daily activities.

⋏ MACS describes how children usually use their hands to handle objects in the home, school, and community settings (what they do), rather than what is known to be their best capacity.

⋏ In order to obtain knowledge about how a child handles various everyday objects, it is necessary to ask someone who knows the child well, rather than through a specific test.

⋏ The objects the child handles should be considered from an age-related perspective.

⋏ MACS classify a child's overall ability to handle objects, not each hand separately.

Information for users

The Manual Ability Classification System (MACS) describes how children with cerebral palsy (CP) use their hands to handle objects in daily activities. MACS describes five levels. The levels are based on the children's self-initiated ability to handle objects and their need for assistance or adaptation to perform manual activities in everyday life. The MACS brochure also describes differences between adjacent levels to make it easier to determine which level best corresponds with the child's ability to handle objects.

The objects referred to are those that are relevant and age-appropriate for the children, used when they perform tasks such as eating, dressing, playing, drawing or writing. It is objects that are within the children's personal space that is referred to, as oppose to objects that are beyond their reach. Objects used in advanced activities that require special skills, such as playing an instrument are not included in this considerations.

When establishing a child's MACS level, choose the level that best describes the child's overall usual performance, in the home, school or community setting. The child's motivation and cognitive ability also affect the ability to handle objects and accordingly influence the MACS level. In order to obtain knowledge about how a child handles various everyday objects it is necessary to ask someone who knows the child well. MACS is intended to classify what the children usually do, not their best possible performance in a specific test situation.

MACS is a functional description that can be used in a way that is complement to the diagnosis of cerebral palsy and its subtypes. MACS assesses the children's overall ability to handle everyday objects, not the function of each hand separately. MACS does not take into account differences in function between the two hands; rather, it addresses how the children handle age-appropriate objects. MACS does not intend to explain the underlying reasons for impaired manual abilities.

MACS can be used for children aged 4–18 years, but certain concepts must be placed in relation to the child's age. Naturally there is a difference in which objects a four-year old should be able to handle, compared with a teenager. The same applies to independence –a young child needs more help and supervision than an older child.

MACS spans the entire spectrum of functional limitations found among children with cerebral palsy and covers all sub-diagnoses. Certain sub-diagnoses can be found at all MACS levels, such as bilateral CP, while others are found at fewer levels, such as unilateral CP. Level I includes children with minor limitations, while children with severe functional limitations will usually be found at levels IV and V. If typically developed children were to be classified according to MACS, however, a level "0" would be needed.

Moreover, each level includes children with relatively varied function. It is unlikely that MACS is sensitive to changes after an intervention; in all probability, MACS levels are stable over time.

The five levels in MACS form an ordinal scale, which means that the levels are 'ordered' but differences between levels are not necessarily equal, nor are children with cerebral palsy equally distributed across the five levels.

E-mail:ann-christin.eliasson@ki.se; www.macs.nu

Eliasson AC, Krumlinde Sundholm L, Rösblad B, Beckung E, Arner M, Öhrvall AM, Rosenbaum P. The Manual Ability Classification System (MACS) for children with cerebral palsy: scale development and evidence of validity and reliability Developmental Medicine and Child Neurology 2006 48:549-554

Available at www.macs.nu

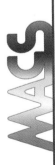

What do you need to know to use MACS?

The child's ability to handle objects in important daily activities, for example during play and leisure, eating and dressing.

In which situation is the child independent and to what extent do they need support and adaptation?

I. **Handles objects easily and successfully.** At most, limitations in the ease of performing manual tasks requiring speed and accuracy. However, any limitations in manual abilities do not restrict independence in daily activities.

II. **Handles most objects but with somewhat reduced quality and/or speed of achievement.** Certain activities may be avoided or be achieved with some difficulty; alternative ways of performance might be used but manual abilities do not usually restrict independence in daily activities.

III. **Handles objects with difficulty; needs help to prepare and/or modify activities.** The performance is slow and achieved with limited success regarding quality and quantity. Activities are performed independently if they have been set up or adapted.

IV. **Handles a limited selection of easily managed objects in adapted situations.** Performs parts of activities with effort and with limited success. Requires continuous support and assistance and/or adapted equipment, for even partial achievement of the activity.

V. **Does not handle objects and has severely limited ability to perform even simple actions.** Requires total assistance.

Distinctions between Levels I and II

Children in Level I may have limitations in handling very small, heavy or fragile objects which demand detailed fine motor control, or efficient coordination between hands. Limitations may also involve performance in new and unfamiliar situations. Children in Level II perform almost the same activities as children in Level I but the quality of performance is decreased, or the performance is slower. Functional differences between hands can limit effectiveness of performance. Children in Level II commonly try to simplify handling of objects, for example by using a surface for support instead of handling objects with both hands.

Distinctions between Levels II and III

Children in Level II handle most objects, although slowly or with reduced quality of performance. Children in Level III commonly need help to prepare the activity and/or require adjustments to be made to the environment since their ability to reach or handle objects is limited. They cannot perform certain activities and their degree of independence is related to the supportiveness of the environmental context.

Distinctions between Levels III and IV

Children in Level III can perform selected activities if the situation is prearranged and if they get supervision and plenty of time. Children in Level IV need continuous help during the activity and can at best participate meaningfully in only parts of an activity.

Distinctions between Levels IV and V

Children in Level IV perform part of an activity, however, they need help continuously. Children in Level V might at best participate with a simple movement in special situations, e.g. by pushing a button or occasionally hold undemanding objects.

Supplementary MACS level identification chart
To be used together with the MACS leaflet

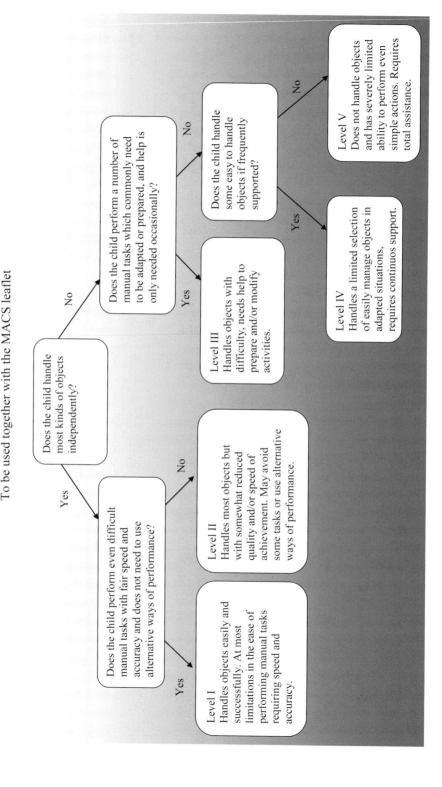

Does the child handle most kinds of objects independently?

Yes

Does the child perform even difficult manual tasks with fair speed and accuracy and does not need to use alternative ways of performance?

Yes

Level I
Handles objects easily and successfully. At most limitations in the ease of performing manual tasks requiring speed and accuracy.

No

Level II
Handles most objects but with somewhat reduced quality and/or speed of achievement. May avoid some tasks or use alternative ways of performance.

No

Does the child perform a number of manual tasks which commonly need to be adapted or prepared, and help is only needed occasionally?

Yes

Level III
Handles objects with difficulty, needs help to prepare and/or modify activities.

No

Does the child handle some easy to handle objects if frequently supported?

Yes

Level IV
Handles a limited selection of easily manage objects in adapted situations, requires continuos support.

No

Level V
Does not handle objects and has severely limited ability to perform even simple actions. Requires total assistance.

Field trial version

196

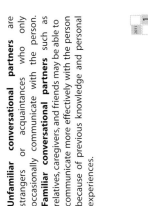

Communication Function Classification System (CFCS) for Individuals with Cerebral Palsy

Purpose

The **purpose** of the CFCS is to classify the **everyday communication performance** of an individual with cerebral palsy into one of five levels. The CFCS focuses on activity and participation levels as described in the World Health Organization's (WHO) International Classification of Functioning, Disability, and Health (ICF).

User Instructions

A parent, caregiver, and/or a professional who is familiar with the person's communication selects the level of communication performance. Adults and adolescents with cerebral palsy may also classify their communication performance. The **overall effectiveness** of the communication performance **should be based on how they usually take part in everyday situations requiring communication,** rather than their best capacity. These everyday situations may occur in home, school, and the community.

Some communication may be difficult to classify if performance falls across more than one level. In those cases, choose the level that **most closely describes** the person's usual performance **in the most settings.** Do not consider the individual's perceived capacity, cognition, and/or motivation when selecting a level.

Definitions

Communication occurs when a **sender** transmits a message **_and_** a **receiver** understands the message. An **effective communicator** independently **alternates as a sender and a receiver** regardless of the demands of a conversation, including settings (e.g., community, school, work, home), conversational partners, and topics.

All methods of communication performance are considered in determining the CFCS level. These include the use of speech, gestures, behaviors, eye gaze, facial expressions, and augmentative and alternative communication (**AAC**). AAC systems include (but are not limited to) manual sign, pictures, communication boards, communication books, and talking devices – sometimes called voice output communication aids (VOCAs) or speech generating devices (SGDs).

Distinctions between the levels are based on the performance of **sender and receiver roles,** the **pace of communication,** and the **type of conversational partner.** The following definitions should be kept in mind when using this classification system.

Effective senders and receivers shift quickly and easily between transmitting and understanding messages. To clarify or repair misunderstandings, the effective sender and receiver may use or request strategies such as repeating, rephrasing, simplifying, and/or expanding the message. To speed up communication exchanges, especially when using AAC, an effective sender may appropriately decide to use less grammatically correct messages by leaving out or shortening words with familiar communication partners.

A **comfortable pace** of communication refers to how quickly and easily the person can understand and convey messages. A comfortable pace occurs with few communication breakdowns and little wait time between communication turns.

Unfamiliar conversational partners are strangers or acquaintances who only occasionally communicate with the person. **Familiar conversational partners** such as relatives, caregivers, and friends may be able to communicate more effectively with the person because of previous knowledge and personal experiences.

Available at http://cfcs.us.

Appendix IV

Examples of growth charts comparing weight for different degrees of severity of CP (GMFCS levels I, II, IV and V). Further charts can be found at http://LifeExpectancy.org?Articles/NewGrowthCharts.shtm.

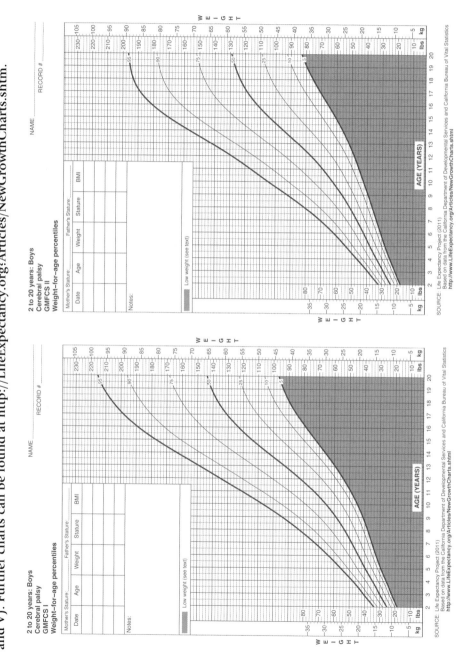

2 to 20 years: Boys
Cerebral palsy
GMFCS I
Weight-for-age percentiles

NAME _____ RECORD # _____

2 to 20 years: Boys
Cerebral palsy
GMFCS II
Weight-for-age percentiles

NAME _____ RECORD # _____

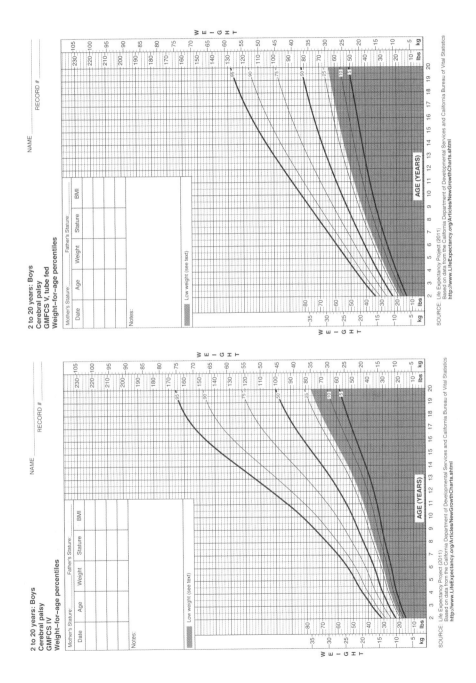

2 to 20 years: Boys
Cerebral palsy
GMFCS IV
Weight–for–age percentiles

Mother's Stature:		Father's Stature:		
Date	Age	Weight	Stature	BMI

Notes:

Low weight (see text)

AGE (YEARS)

W E I G H T

SOURCE: Life Expectancy Project (2011)
Based on data from the California Department of Developmental Services and California Bureau of Vital Statistics
http://www.LifeExpectancy.org/Articles/NewGrowthCharts.shtml

NAME _____ RECORD # _____

2 to 20 years: Boys
Cerebral palsy
GMFCS V, tube fed
Weight–for–age percentiles

Mother's Stature:		Father's Stature:		
Date	Age	Weight	Stature	BMI

Notes:

Low weight (see text)

AGE (YEARS)

W E I G H T

SOURCE: Life Expectancy Project (2011)
Based on data from the California Department of Developmental Services and California Bureau of Vital Statistics
http://www.LifeExpectancy.org/Articles/NewGrowthCharts.shtml

NAME _____ RECORD # _____

199

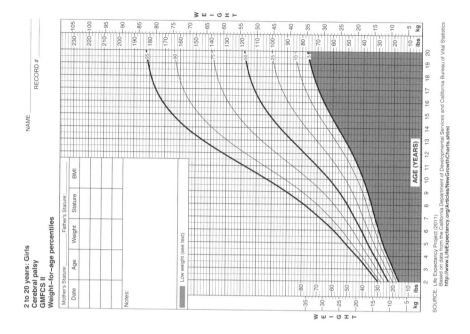

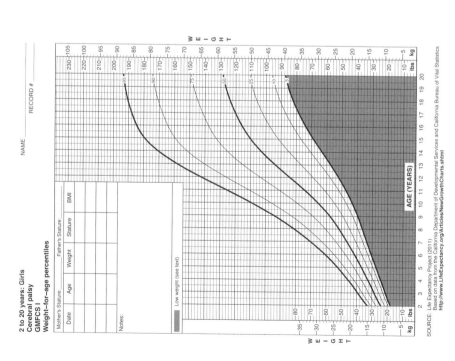

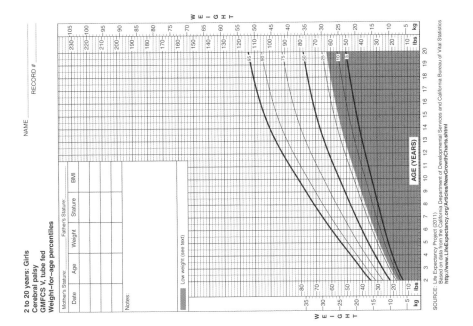

2 to 20 years: Girls
Cerebral palsy
GMFCS IV
Weight–for–age percentiles

NAME _____ RECORD # _____

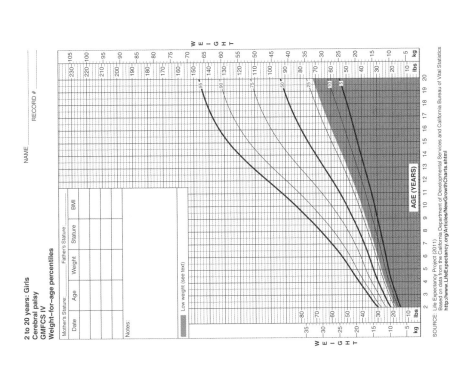

2 to 20 years: Girls
Cerebral palsy
GMFCS V, tube fed
Weight–for–age percentiles

NAME _____ RECORD # _____

201

Appendix V

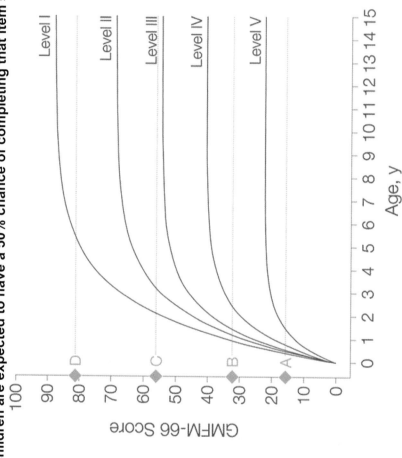

Predicted Average Motor Development by the Gross Motor Function Classification System Levels. The diamonds on the vertical axis identify 4 Gross Motor Function Measure-66 (GMFM-66) items that predict when children are expected to have a 50% chance of completing that item successfully.

Rosenbaum, P. L. et al. JAMA 2002;288:1357-1363

JAMA

Index

Notes

Page number in *italics* refer to material in tables or figures. vs indicates a comparison or differential diagnosis.

The following abbreviation has been used:
CP, cerebral palsy